The Fit-or-Fat Target Diet

COVERT BAILEY

SPHERE BOOKS LIMITED
London and Sydney

First published in the United States of America
by Houghton Mifflin Company 1984
First published in Great Britain by
Sphere Books Ltd 1986
30–32 Gray's Inn Road, London WC1X 8JL
Copyright © 1984 by Covert Bailey

Publisher's Note

This edition has been thoroughly revised,
with Imperial and metric measurements throughout.

TRADE
MARK

Set in Times

Printed and bound in Great Britain by
Cox & Wyman Ltd, Reading

This book is dedicated to Lea

Contents

1

Diets Don't Work

We are obsessed with diets! Fat people want to lose weight. Doctors search for ways to reduce salt and cholesterol. Runners hunt for foods that give them lasting energy. Parents worry about junk foods. All of us – fit or fat – are concerned about the quality of our food. It seems as though a new diet is written every ten minutes. Pick up any magazine and you're sure to see the latest quick-weight-loss scheme – usually endorsed by a favourite Hollywood personality. Many new diets claim a prestigious origin such as Cambridge or Harvard. Yet our mania for diets doesn't seem to be working, because we are getting fatter all the time. It seems the more we go on diets, the fatter we get. The steady rise in obesity, coupled with the wild proliferation of diet books, tells me one thing – diets don't work!

Why, then, did I name this book *The Fit-or-Fat Target Diet*? Because it *is* concerned with food: how to buy it, prepare it and eat it. There is even a chapter on how to lose weight. But the Target Diet is not a diet. It's a system for evaluating foods, diets and menus. It doesn't say to eat this on Monday and that on Tuesday. It doesn't say this food is forbidden while that food is a must. It *does*, however, give a framework – a system for you to use in evaluating any diet. Suppose, for example, you question the wisdom of vegetarian eating. In Chapter 7, the foods a foolish vegetarian might choose are analysed, using the Target system, so you can see why we call him a dumb vegetarian. Chapter 8 again uses the Target to analyse the food choices of a smart vegetarian.

To many people, the word *diet* means a low-calorie, highly regimented weight-loss programme. To others, *diet* means temporary misery until some medical problem is resolved. The Target Diet is none of these. It is merely a system that allows you to evaluate for yourself the wisdom or folly of any dietary scheme.

Dietitians will like the Target approach because their patients will better understand nutritional advice. Doctors will use it because there isn't anything far-out or quacky about it. And *you* will like it because it will give you the power to make your own nutritional analysis. It will allow you to eat wisely, tailoring your diet to your own personal tastes and requirements. The Target Diet can help the marathon runner who wants 4000 high-carbohydrate calories, and it can also help the fat executive find adequate protein and vitamins in just 1700 calories. Best of all, once you learn the system, it will last you a lifetime.

2

Fat in the Diet – Number One Enemy

Nutrition is complicated – it's hard to know where to start. I may have prejudiced you already by the title of this chapter. You may feel that fat is *not* the worst thing in our diet. Bear with me, and I'm sure I can change your mind.

Nutritionists consult tables to look up the ingredients in a food. These tables give the number of calories in a serving of a food and also show how many of those calories come from fat. If you check a few of your favourite foods, you will probably be shocked. In peanuts, for example, 75 per cent of the calories comes from fat. People think of nuts as high-protein foods, whereas, in fact, they contain a lot of fat and very little protein. Most men can eat a handful of peanuts without a second thought. A handful of peanuts is about 3½ oz (100 g) and contains 566 calories, of which 325 come from fat.

1 gram of fat	= 9 calories
1 gram of protein	= 4 calories
1 gram of carbohydrate	= 4 calories

We get more than double the calories from the fat we eat than we do from the protein or carbohydrate. Or another way to put it is that a small amount of fatty food contains more calories than a large amount of lean food.

Meat, nuts and milk products tend to be very high in fat in addition to being a bit expensive. The result is that affluent nations are full of fat people. Financially, we can afford to eat expensive but greasy foods. Fat in our diet is making us fat because one can get an awful lot of calories out of a small amount of food. Fat people are prone to heart attack, diabetes, kidney disease, gallbladder problems and a host of other medical conditions. Fat people fill our hospitals. Obesity is our number one health problem, making fat our number one nutritional enemy.

Don't overreact to this statement by reminding me that we need some fat in the diet. I am well aware that we need oleic and linoleic acids, that fat provides a satiety (fullness) factor, and that fat carries the fat-soluble vitamins. The point is that you would have to go to extremes to eat a fat-deficient diet because fat is hidden in foods where you would never suspect it to be. You certainly won't suffer any ill effects from fat deprivation if you follow the Target rules presented in the following chapters.

Don't make the mistake of thinking that one kind of fat is okay but another is not – that polyunsaturated fats are good but saturated fats are bad. Recent evidence indicates that the kind of fat you eat – beef fat, butter fat or vegetable oils – isn't the critical issue. The important thing is to eat less of it.

A large baked potato has only 139 calories. Add ½ oz (15 g) of butter and it jumps to 246 calories. Add another ½ oz (15 g) of butter and a little soured cream, and you may have 380 calories. At that point the potato itself is only 37 per cent of the total calories. It's too bad that so many people blame the potato for being the fattening food.

Some people eliminate all red meats, feeling that they can then eat more nuts. That just replaces one fat food with another. Others are proud that they have replaced butter, which is 100 per cent fat, with margarine – which is also 100 per cent fat! I often tease my audiences that putting butter or margarine on food is the same as pouring on a little motor oil or smearing on some Vaseline; they're all 100 per cent grease.

The medical effects of a high-fat diet are devastating. Arteriosclerosis, high blood cholesterol and triglycerides, and even cancer of the colon have been linked to high fat consumption. If these ailments do not concern you and all you really want is a slim figure, then decrease the fat in your diet anyway. You need no other reason than the awful number of calories that fats contain. It doesn't matter too much how you do it, but get the fat out.

3

What Is a Balanced Diet?

To achieve a perfect diet, you need obey only four rules:

1. Be sure to eat a balanced diet.
2. Select foods that are low in fat.
3. Select foods that are low in sugar.
4. Select foods that are high in fibre.

If you follow these rules, you needn't worry about cholesterol, saturated fats, vitamins, trace minerals, or most of today's other nutritional concerns. You don't even have to worry about preservatives or other additives in food. In short, observe the four basic rules, and the rest comes without asking.

Balancing the diet is the rule most often neglected, but it is the most important one, because it underlies every other nutritional consideration. We must eat a variety of foods in order to be certain that we get the full variety of nutrients. This seems like common sense to most of us, for we know that different foods provide different elements. Therefore, be suspicious when claims are made about the extraordinary effects of any one food. Don't believe the articles that claim peanut butter cures depression or that gelatine stimulates nail growth. In fact, diets that emphasise one group of foods or just one food should be discarded immediately.

No single food or group of foods contains everything we need. So, taking the more level-headed approach, we should eat from a wide selection of foods. The idea has so much merit that one might be tempted to go to the opposite extreme. After all, if one aspirin is good, then two must be better; a person might try to eat every food that exists in order not to miss some elusive trace mineral. The idea gets pretty ridiculous when we imagine the thousands of foods available in the world, including chocolate-covered ants, rattlesnake meat and weird foreign vegetables that most of us have never heard of. It would not only be impossible to eat every food, but many foods should be left out because they do more harm than good. Best of all, it isn't necessary, because we can group foods according to their nutrient content, as examplified by the 'Four-Food Groups', the 'Seven-Food Groups' systems and a dozen lesser-known food-grouping systems.

In the United States it was found convenient to divide foods into four groups, but nutritionists working in rural India found that people simply couldn't grasp the reason for four groups. They also found that food was too scarce for the people to be *able* to select from four groups. So the nutritionists divided foods into only two groups – the High-Protein Group and the Low-Protein Group. Some scientists criticised this approach on the grounds that food selections from just two groups can often be inadequate. They were scientifically correct, but they weren't aware of the difficulties inherent in teaching people who know very little and have very little to choose from.

In some rural cultures, a Three-Food-Group system has been used, in which the high-protein foods are further divided into those that come from meat (flesh or lentils, peas and beans) and those that come from milk. This gives us the Meat Group, the Milk Group and the Low-Protein Group.

In the United States we further divide the Low-Protein Group into the Fruit and Vegetable Group and the Bread and Cereal (Grain) Group, yielding the Four-Food Groups.

One could carry this sorting process another step by dividing the fruits and vegetables. After all, the nutrient content of fruits (predominantly vitamin C) is quite different from that supplied by vegetables (predominantly vitamin A). This would yield five food groups. The Weight Watchers organisation (to its credit) goes one step further, dividing the vegetables into a low-calorie group and a high-calorie group, yielding six food groups.

In the 1960s, nutritionists thought that essential fatty acids were so important that they added still another group (which isn't really a group of foods at all) called essential fats or oils. This gave rise to the Seven-Food-Group system that was then taught in most nutrition and home economics classes. Today we know that these essential fatty acids are bountifully present in practically every food, so it isn't necessary to make a special group for them. In fact, we are so down on fats that we shudder at this former emphasis. It's almost impossible to get too little fat or too few essential fatty acids, no matter how poor one's food selections.

This business of dividing foods into groups has been carried to ridiculous extremes by nutritionists in Colombia, who evolved an Eleven-Food-Group system. No one (including yours truly) was able to remember them all.

In the Four-Food Group system, eggs are classified in the Meat Group because they contain the protein, vitamins and minerals of meat. The uninitiated put eggs in the Milk Group because they are white and are found next to the milk products in the supermarket. We must be careful not to classify foods by colour, where they grow, or where we buy them. It's what is *in* the food that matters. Green peas are classified in the Vegetable Group because their outstanding nutrient is vitamin A. But if peas are allowed to remain on the vine as the plant matures and dies, they take on some of the characteristics of seeds, all of which

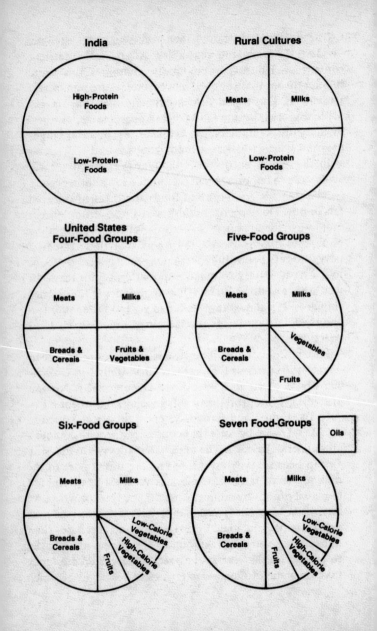

India

High-Protein Foods

Low-Protein Foods

Rural Cultures

Meats

Milks

Low-Protein Foods

**United States
Four-Food Groups**

Meats

Milks

Breads & Cereals

Fruits & Vegetables

Five-Food Groups

Meats

Milks

Breads & Cereals

Vegetables

Fruits

Six-Food Groups

Meats

Milks

Breads & Cereals

Low-Calorie Vegetables

High-Calorie Vegetables

Fruits

Seven Food-Groups

Oils

Meats

Milks

Breads & Cereals

Low-Calorie Vegetables

High-Calorie Vegetables

Fruits

are high in protein, iron and niacin. So split peas go in the Meat Group, even though they are vegetables by birthright. If you are wondering how to classify a food, think about what's *in* the food, not where it grows. People put potatoes in the 'starch' group, which isn't even a legitimate group. In fact, potatoes are very low in calories and high in vitamin C, so they are properly put in the Fruit and Vegetable Group. Corn on the cob seems at first to be a vegetable, but in reality it's a tall grain classified with rice, wheat, rye and other grains.

I am amazed by those who think they are nutrition-conscious but cannot name the main nutrients of each food group. Such people are so concerned with exotic vitamins that they overlook the fact that all the vitamins, even the exotic ones, are found in food – *if* one eats a great variety of foods. If you can't name the main nutrients – that is, the three primary nutrients of each food group – but you can tell me all the latest news about vitamin E or bran, you are kidding yourself – you haven't even learned the basics. What good is it to study the supposed wonders of bran if you don't even know that those wonders come from cellulose fibre, one of the prime ingredients of the breads and cereals?

Leader Nutrients of Each Food Group

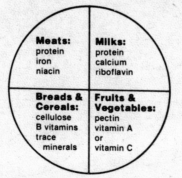

Meats:
protein
iron
niacin

Milks:
protein
calcium
riboflavin

Breads & Cereals:
cellulose
B vitamins
trace
   minerals

Fruits & Vegetables:
pectin
vitamin A
or
vitamin C

Memorise these rules:

1. To be classified in the Meat Group, a food must contain significant quantities of protein, iron and niacin (vitamin B3).

2. Milk-Group foods must contain significant quantities of protein, calcium and riboflavin (vitamin B2).

3. Fruits and vegetables must contain pectin fibre, plus either vitamin A or vitamin C.

4. Breads and cereals must contain significant quantities of cellulose fibre, plus B vitamins and trace minerals.

The Bread and Cereal Group has the least specific definition and is the most maligned by fat people, yet it is the survival food for three-quarters of the world's population. Not only do the poor people of the world exist on grain products, but they have little of the heart disease, obesity, or arteriosclerosis that plague us. They must be doing something right! In the West we have come to think of bread as poor man's food and thick steaks as symbolising the good life. The truth is that a mouthful of steak is about five times as fattening as a mouthful of good bread.

4

The Target Concept

I use the Four-Food-Group system as the basis of my Target Diet because it satisfies the most fundamental of my four basic rules – eat a balanced diet.

To help illustrate the other three rules (low-fat, low-sugar, high-fibre), inner circles are added to the Four-Food-Group circle, making it into a Target (see page 15). Then, focusing on one food group at a time, foods are graded until the best ones in that group are in the centre of the Target and the worst selections are on the periphery. All the foods above the centre line (the meats and milks) are graded according to their fat content.

In the Milk Group, fluid milk is the quickest and easiest to classify. Skimmed (or nonfat) milk goes in the centre ring, since it has no fat at all. One per cent fat milk is next to the skimmed; 2 per cent, or low-fat, in the next ring; whole milk, which is 3.5 per cent, is in the outer ring. Ice cream is so high in fat that we put it outside the Target. Butter, like lard, margarine and mayonnaise, is pure fat containing virtually no vitamins, minerals or protein. Butter isn't a food at all – it's grease extracted from a food called milk.

The amounts of fat in the other dairy products are a little less obvious. Low-fat yoghurt, commercial buttermilk, and low-fat cottage cheese are made from skimmed milk (or very close to it), so they fall in the centre of the circle. Part-skim mozzarella cheese falls in the next circle, and cheddar cheese, like most cheeses, in the third circle. (It seems as if all the cheeses I like go in the third circle.)

Note that whole milk, at 3.5 per cent fat, falls in the same ring as cheddar cheese. Fluid milk is about 85 per cent water, 3.5 per cent fat, and the remaining 11.5 per cent is protein and carbohydrate. Of the total 160 calories in a glass of milk, 50 per cent comes from fat. In other words, fat may be only 3.5 per cent of the volume of a glass of milk, but it supplies 50 per cent of the calories.

The Meat Group is also separated according to fat content, with beans and other legumes located at the bull's-eye. A simple definition of a legume is anything that grows in a pea type of pod. That includes split peas, garbanzo or chick peas, lentils, black-eyed beans, haricot beans, and dozens more. Note that peanuts grow underground, not hanging in a pod, so they don't go in the bull's-eye. Peanuts and peanut butter are nutritious, but because they are very fatty, they are placed in the third ring, with beef. Even dry-roasted peanuts are 79 per cent fat calories. Most nuts are even fattier than peanuts, so they parallel many cuts of beef. Tuna packed in brine, like beans, is less than 10 per cent fat, whereas salmon is about 59 per cent fat calories. Obviously, you can't assume that all fish is low in fat.

Most pork products are so high in fat that I place them just outside the outer ring, parallel to ice cream in the Milk Group. I put suet on the diagram mostly for fun, but you should keep in mind that suet is pure grease separated from meat, just as butter is pure grease extracted from milk. Butter just happens to have an awful lot of flavour.

I hope that at this point you are eager to ask me where on the Target to put lobster, venison or liver. There are hundreds of meats and dairy products that we will have to place correctly, but first let's just get the principle of the Target Diet. In later chapters, I will deal with more specifics and show you how to make the Target work for you. For now, let's look at the foods below the centre line of the Target.

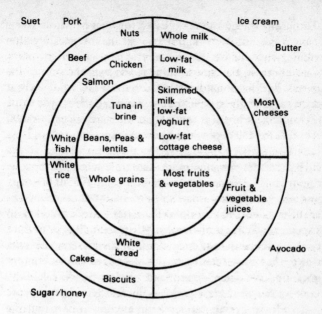

Everything below the centre line is a plant product (the animal products – plus nuts and beans – being above the line), graded by its fibre content, which you can think of as its 'wholeness', or 'whole-grainness', or how close it is to its natural state when eaten. Cake is made of wheat flour, just as wholemeal bread is, but wholemeal flour is much closer to the natural wheat than highly refined white cake flour.

In the Bread and Cereal Group, whole grains go in the bull's-eye. Whole grain means unrefined, unground, unbleached – in short, untouched. One can still buy honest-to-goodness whole wheat. Bran, which is so highly touted for its fibre content, is nothing but the chaff, or husk, or outside covering of wheat, similar to the husk on an ear of corn. You can eat bran after it has been removed from wheat or you can eat whole wheat. I urge people to eat the whole wheat because the trace mineral content is higher.

The bran, wheat and germ eaten together as whole wheat have more nutrition than if you eat them separately after refinement. The whole is greater than the sum of the parts.

In contrast, the caloric value is *less than* the sum of the parts. The bran naturally attached to the whole wheat decreases the digestibility of the starch, so the caloric value of wholemeal bread is lower than the charts usually show. About 1 lb (450 g) of white bread has more calories and less nutrition than 1 lb (450 g) of wholemeal bread because the carbohydrate becomes more digestible when the bran is removed. The same is true for rice, corn, rye, millet, oats and any other grain you can think of. About 4 oz (125 g) cornflour will make you a lot fatter than 6 oz (175 g) sweetcorn. What a shame it is that we deliberately alter cereal grains so that the vitamin/mineral content goes down, the fibre content goes down, and the caloric content goes up. We seem determined to destroy ourselves by making our foods less and less nutritious.

To a lesser degree, refinement is also destructive to fruits and vegetables. When fruits or vegetables are made into juices, the effectiveness of the fibre is decreased. Note also that juices are quite high in sugar, because it takes a lot of fruit or vegetable to make a little juice. This is also true of dried fruits. One bunch of grapes might satisfy you, but when those grapes are dried into raisins, they become so small that you want to eat more. We tend to eat more actual fruit in the dried form, therefore getting more sugar. A few years ago, it was fashionable to make juices out of everything. Innumerable juice bars appeared catering for the 'health food' enthusiasts. Some of my students were into the juices and the protein drinks, saying they were far-out. They were far-out all right – far-out on the dietary target!

In the Bread and Cereal Group, whole unrefined grains go in the bull's-eye; they include wholemeal bread, rolled oats cereal, sweetcorn and Shredded Wheat. The first ring outside the bull's-eye contains white bread, white rice, raisin bran and muesli. Note that as grains (particularly wheat) are further refined, sugar is usually added. As we move away from the centre of the Bread and Cereal Group, the vitamin/mineral content goes down, the fibre content goes down, the sugar content goes up, and usually the fat content goes up. Cake recipes call for some fat, and biscuit recipes call for a lot of fat.

The last food group – Fruits and Vegetables – is the easiest to discuss because almost all fruits and vegetables are low in fat, low in calories and high in fibre. Practically all of them go in the bull's-eye, unless you simply extract juice from them. Avocados and olives are so full of fat that we have to put them on the periphery.

It should be obvious that very fat people should eat from the bull's-eye only. The less fat individual can add the next ring of food, and the *very fit* can get away with limited peripheral selections.

If you and I could get our children and our friends to read this chapter and then make more of their food selections from the bull's-eye, we would bring about 90 per cent of the dietary change that is needed. The myriad books on bran, mixing and matching proteins and vitamin supplements are superfluous. If people would live by the rules of this chapter, we could stop here. The rest of the book will convince you that what I am saying is true and will suggest some easy ways to make the changes.

5

The Target Diet –
Fringe Benefits

In this chapter I want to explain how adherence to the Target Diet will satisfy most of the other legitimate nutritional concerns of the day.

The Target on pages 62–63 has been expanded to include many more foods.

Note that cholesterol is found only in animal fats and therefore only in peripheral foods of the Meat and Milk groups. As we move towards the centre of the Target, cholesterol decreases. Bull's-eye foods have no cholesterol at all and, of course, these are the foods that heart patients are urged to eat. The one exception to this is the shellfish, which are located near the centre of the Target because of their low-fat content but which are somewhat high in cholesterol. Bacon and ice cream are so high in fat and in cholesterol content that they are no-nos for anyone with heart disease. What a shame it is that we continue to eat high-cholesterol foods, slowly closing our arteries, and then think about making dietary changes when the damage has been done. A nice fringe benefit of the Target Diet is that it doesn't require the eater to *think* about cholesterol, because a diet that is low in fat is automatically low in cholesterol. The American Heart Association has urged a low-cholesterol diet for years but, typically, only those at high risk have paid much attention. The Target approach should appeal to everyone, for it provides a low-cholesterol diet even for one who isn't particularly concerned about it.

The American Heart Association has also urged us to switch emphasis from saturated (animal) fats to poly-unsaturated (vegetable) fats. I think we should decrease *total* fat and not worry about what kind. Unfortunately, people were led to believe that polyunsaturated fats (oils, actually) were *good* for us; what the Heart Association meant was that they were *less bad* for us. The result was that lots of people gave up butter but increased their total fat intake by using large amounts of margarine instead. I prefer the Target approach – decrease the total fat in your diet. If the total dietary fat is low enough, the type of fat becomes relatively insignificant.

Another advantage of the Target is that the intake of food additives is automatically reduced. This is parti-cularly obvious in the breads and cereals. Packaged cakes, biscuits and pastries contain staggering amounts of preservatives. Food dyes, stabilisers, texturisers, flavour enhancers – you name it – they all show up in the packaged sugar-rich, fibre-poor breads and cereals. The more natural and fibre-rich the grain product, the fewer the additives. In the meats and milks, food additives rise as the fat level goes up. So as one moves towards the centre of the Target, the purity of the foods increases, producing another health spin-off of low-fat, low-sugar, high-fibre eating.

Perhaps the greatest advantage of eating from the centre of the Target is the sharp increase in the nutrient content, sometimes called nutrient density. Be aware, however, that there are several ways of reporting nutrient density. One of these methods lists the vitamin/mineral content per spoonful or, more typically, per serving, and this is grossly misleading. For example, when cereals are graded on their nutrient content per serving, they end up looking quite poor. Fruits and vegetables also show low ratings. Several years ago a rather sensational report appeared in which cereals were rated by their vitamin/mineral content per serving. By this method some of the natural whole-grain cereals looked worse than those that were highly refined and filled with sugar. The refined, fibre-poor cereals, fortified with vitamins and minerals, were made to look great on the label, but their lack of fibre and protein was obscured, as was their sugar calorie content. If all you report is the vitamin/mineral content of a food, a bowl of stewed apples looks very poor next to a serving of beef. In other words, based on nutrients *per serving*, the meat looks much better. However, the beef has many more calories.

Listing vitamins/minerals/protein *per calorie* of a food is the sensible way to evaluate nutrient density. In Scandinavia, food labels include a diagram that neatly illustrates this second method. No numbers are used; instead, there is simply a circle with a section at the top like a piece of pie, which get bigger if a food is rich in vitamins/minerals, and a piece of pie at the bottom, representing the calorie content. Obviously, the best foods would have large sections at the top and small sections at the bottom. Tuna in brine, which contains lots of vitamins, minerals and protein per calorie, would look something like the diagram below. Salami, on the other hand, would

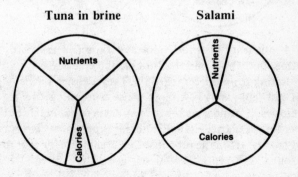

Tuna in brine   **Salami**

21

go way out on the periphery of the Target because of its incredibly high fat count and its low vitamin/mineral content.

On the Target, the nutrients per calorie rise as one approaches the bull's-eye. It's true that a glass of whole milk contains the same amount of vitamin/mineral/protein as a glass of skimmed milk, but the whole milk contains double the calories because of its fat content. In the old days, whole milk was considered nutritious because it contains many nutrients. In the new sense, whole milk isn't nutritious, because its nutrition per calorie is too low. If you drink 2 glasses of skimmed milk, you get the same number of calories as from 1 glass of whole, but you get twice the vitamins, minerals and protein.

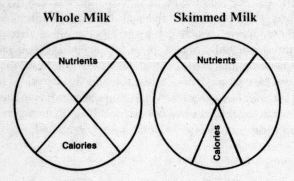

The nutrients in whole milk and skimmed milk are the same, but whole milk has double the calories.

Eating from the centre of the Target ensures a diet high in nutrient density without your consuming too many calories. If – and it's a big if – you eat predominately bull's-eye foods, taking vitamin/mineral supplements is a waste of money. If, on the other hand, you eat from the four food groups but your selections are white bread, fried courgettes, whole milk and bacon, you will not only be vitamin/mineral deficient but you will also get fat! As you get fatter, you may decide to eat less, but if you continue to make the same poor selections, you'll get progressively fewer and fewer vitamins and minerals. The people in the United States who have marginal vitamin deficiencies don't have them because foods are grown on poor soil or because of slow shipping or handling. They're caused by the low-nutrient-density, high-fat, high-sugar foods that they eat. That puts the blame where it belongs – not on the farmer, the food handlers, or the markets, but squarely on the eater!

There are several other spin-off advantages to the Target. Foods at the centre tend to be low in salt (although this advantage can easily be negated at the dinner table). Bull's-eye foods usually cost less, and food prices are high enough to make the economy of Target foods important to all of us. Foods from the centre of the Target are often easily stored. Reasonably edible whole wheat was found in King Tut's tomb, and edible potatoes have been found that were buried with the Inca Indians. Beans simply stored in bags are known to last for years. People in the poorer countries without modern refrigeration and storage facilities owe their existence to the grains, peas and beans.

I started this whole discussion of the Target Diet by claiming that one need obey only four dietary rules. You can now see that the Target Diet, based on these four rules, actually provides for most of today's other dietary requisites as well, for it is:

● low in fat	● low in saturated fats
● low in sugar	● low in cost
● low in calories	● highly storable
● low in salt	● high in fibre
● low in additives	● high in nutrient density
● low in cholesterol	● a balanced diet

I like the Target Diet best of all because it allows me to eat a lot of food, thus satisfying my desire to 'stuff' myself. For the same number of calories, I can have 16 fl oz (450 ml) skimmed milk instead of 8 fl oz (250 ml) of whole. A big bowl of split-pea soup and some wholemeal bread have the same number of calories but satisfy me more than a 3½ oz (100 g) hamburger. I can have four or five oranges instead of 1 glass of orange juice. I find that whole-grain bread fills me up more quickly and stops my hunger longer than a packet of biscuits. This is one diet that doesn't ask me to go hungry. I am able to eat any foods I happen to enjoy, as long as they are near the centre of the Target. In fact, once you get used to the Target Diet, you will have no feeling of denial at all.

6

Practical Ways to Get the Fat out of Your Diet

I find myself at a large group lunch or dinner two or three times a week. I can't help observing other people's food choices. They typically avoid the 'starchy' foods, such as potatoes and bread, while putting scoops of dressing on their salads. Or they 'ration' themselves to half a roll but use two pats of butter. They don't seem to realise that an entire baked potato contains fewer calories than 2 tablespoons of salad dressing. The cautious bread eater would be calorically wiser if he ate two rolls and omitted the butter. Moreover, it should be obvious to anyone that the vitamins, minerals and fibre are in the rolls and potatoes, not in the butter or salad dressing.

I can't understand why it's so popular to say that carbohydrates are fattening. *Fat is fattening!* By cutting out fat, you can eat as much as, or more than, usual and yet reduce calorie consumption by 40 to 50 per cent. A very large baked potato has about 140 calories in it. If you make chips from that potato you more than double the calories because of the fat used in frying. Let's look at foods – one food group at a time – and discuss ways of eliminating fats from each group.

Milk Group

I changed from whole milk to skimmed milk by buying 2 pints (1.2 litres) of whole milk and 2 pints (1.2 litres) of 2 per cent low-fat and mixing them. In a few weeks I was able to wean myself away from whole milk and began to enjoy drinking the 2 per cent low-fat milk. Then I combined 2 per cent fat milk with 1 per cent fat until the flavour of the 1 per cent was good by itself. Several months later the same trick worked with 1 per cent fat and skimmed milk. Occasionally, during this 'defatting' process, I would treat myself to some low-fat chocolate milk. True, the sugar in the chocolate milk added to the calories, but I was learning to like skimmed milk at the same time.

Most people are surprised to learn that buttermilk is very low in fat. You can make a tasty low-fat snack by blending it with frozen fruit juice concentrate or frozen fruits like strawberries. Many baking recipes that call for whole milk yield more flavourful and less fattening results when you substitute buttermilk.

It was difficult for me to cut down on cheese consumption. Fortunately, I love cottage cheese, and low-fat cottage cheese substitutes very nicely in many recipes (such as lasagna and omelettes) that call for the higher-fat cheeses. Experiment with Gjetost, Jarlsberg and the new low-fat cheeses on the market – although they are still fairly high in fat (50 per cent) they are considerably lower than Cheddar or Roquefort, at 80 per cent fat, or cream cheese, at 89 per cent fat! I now use the high-fat cheeses as a treat or a garnish rather than a main course. If you love your cream cheese, try the lower-fat Neufchâtel instead. If a recipe calls for cheese, use one with a very sharp flavour – you can use much less and still get the cheesy taste.

I disliked plain yoghurt when I was a child, so I had to employ the same trick that I used with milk to learn to like it. I ate the fruit-flavoured kind (high in sugar but low in fat) until I grew used to the taste. Now I use plain yoghurt quite frequently in salad dressings and vegetable toppings.

There's only one thing that I like better than ice cream.

And that's more ice cream! Unfortunately, it's off my list except for my birthday. Now I have iced milk, sorbet or custard made with skimmed milk as an occasional dessert when I've been exercising more than usual.

Meat Group

Trim the fat off everything! And cut off the fat *before* you cook. People ask if it makes any difference whether you remove the fat before or after the meat is cooked. You bet it does! A dietitian I work with experimented with a couple of equal-sized roasts. Roast number one was trimmed of all visible fat before it was cooked. The trimmed fat yielded 8 fl oz (250 ml) of grease, which is approximately 2000 calories. Roast number two was cooked untrimmed. Only 4 fl oz (120 ml) of grease could be poured off after it was cooked. In other words, 1000 calories of grease soaked into the second roast and couldn't be removed. The same is true for chicken. If you remove the skin from a whole chicken before cooking it, you'll eliminate about 55 per cent of the calories. If you wait until after cooking to remove the skin, then some of the fat has soaked into the meat and you'll cut out only about half as many calories.

Here's a good trick for cooking minced meat. When browning it in a frying pan, put a large spoon under one edge of the pan. Brown the meat in the elevated portion of the pan, allowing the fat to drain off into the lower part. You can take off a lot more fat this way than by trying to spoon it out after it has soaked into the meat.

'Fry' all your meats by roasting them in the oven in a non-stick pan rather than cooking them in fat in a frying-pan. Better yet, try grilling them, or use a wok. You don't need to use oil in a wok; water or stock will do the job just as well.

If you love red meat, stick to such lower-fat cuts as rump

27

steak or veal. Don't make the mistake some vegetarians do of thinking that nuts and seeds are a good substitute for meat. They contain far more fat! A handful of peanuts is about 566 calories and 75 per cent fat; a grilled 3½ oz (100 g) lean steak is about 250 calories and 21 per cent fat. I've cut out nuts entirely. The amounts of protein and pleasure I get from them just aren't worth the calories.

White fish is a good low-fat bargain. Just don't ruin it by frying it in butter or adding rich sauces. Experiment with spices, wine, yoghurt, lemon juice, vegetables, stock or canned soups, and other seasonings to make flavourful low-fat toppings.

Beans and other peas or lentils are the lowest-fat foods you can eat in the Meat Group. When I first started my new low-fat diet, I didn't know anything about beans. I went to the grocer's and bought every kind of dried bean available. On my first attempt, I cooked up some butter beans with some onion, celery and carrots. I admit I approached the brew with some trepidation. It was delicious! I ate the whole potful in one day – and I was ill for a week! Nowadays I don't go overboard on my beans, but they are a staple of my diet. If you like the flavour of meat, add a well-trimmed ham hock or skinned chicken or just plain chicken stock. I like to cook up three or four different kinds of beans, throw in some barley, and with a couple of chicken breasts and some chopped vegetables, I have a meal for a king!

Fruit and Vegetable Group

Most nutritionists applaud the recent popularity of salad bars. Statistics show that Americans and other affluent societies shortchange the Fruit and Vegetable Group the most, and the salad bar is helping tremendously to get this group of foods back into the diet. The problem is that most people impair these nutritious, low-fat, high-fibre foods by adding lashings of greasy dressing. Watching people at a salad bar has convinced me that they like Roquefort dressing more than salad. I would venture a guess that the typical plateful carried from the salad bar contains about 400 calories. And most people go back for seconds! Most of the calories, of course, come from the dressing. Fortunately, a number of restaurants now offer a reduced-calorie dressing among their selections. (By the way, do you know the difference between reduced-calorie and low-calorie food? *Reduced-calorie* means the product must contain at least one-third fewer calories than a similar food that is not reduced, but it must be equal nutritionally to the food for which it is a substitute. *Low-calorie* means that the food contains no more than 40 calories per serving.)

There are several tricks whereby you can have your salad dressing without the high calories. You can order it separately, along with half a glass of milk, and then mix the two so that you have a reduced-calorie dressing. Or you can order oil and vinegar or lemon juice, which are usually brought to your table in separate containers so you can add as little oil as you want. You can also bring your own homemade dressing to the restaurant. Lots of good packaged mixes now on the market use no oil or fat at all. If the package calls for mayonnaise, substitute yoghurt, buttermilk, or low-fat cottage cheese. Buttermilk or skimmed milk are good substitutes when a recipe lists whole milk. I know some people who blend tofu into their dressings with good results.

With the exception of avocados and olives, fruits and vegetables are low in fat. Again, learn how to top them with creative low-fat sauces rather than butter, cream sauces or cheese. A baked potato is great topped with a blend of cottage cheese, chives, Worcestershire sauce and mustard.

I urge people to eat the natural whole fruit or vegetable rather than extracting the juice or drying it. A whole apricot has more fibre and fewer free sugars than a glass of apricot juice. When the apricot is dried, the sugar content is more than doubled. You also get a greater feeling of satiety by eating the whole fruit or vegetable and thus consume fewer calories. One orange will usually satisfy you, but you will often still be hungry after drinking one cup of orange juice (which is made from four to five oranges).

Bread and Cereal Group

Just because bread is dark in colour doesn't mean it's high in fibre. When I say, 'Read the label', I am referring to the list of ingredients – not the title on the package. If it doesn't say 100 per cent whole wheat or whole rye, then it isn't the right stuff. Keep in mind that the more whole grain a product contains, the higher its fibre content. And if the fibre content is high the calories will be low, because the fibre tends to be difficult to digest and 'ties up' many of the calories so that they are not digested and go right through you. The best way to enjoy the grains is to mix them with other foods. Get into the habit of tossing brown rice, bran, barley or bulgur wheat into your soups, casseroles and salads. My breakfast now consists almost entirely of high-fibre cereals, such as Shredded Wheat and bran, topped with stewed apple or a banana and skimmed milk.

In baking, substitute wholemeal pastry flour for white flour. And as a rule of thumb, I've found that you can safely cut the oil and sugar in a recipe by at least one-half without spoiling the flavour. An acquaintance of mine stumbled on this rule quite by chance. Mixing batter for waffles one day, she discovered that she had only 4 tablespoons of oil, and the recipe called for 6 fl oz (175 ml). She made the waffles anyway, and her family never noticed the difference. She has since been able to reduce the oil all the way down to less than 1 tablespoon and still make great waffles. When you reduce the oil in a recipe, be sure to use either a nonstick baking pan or spray the pan with a nonstick product because such baked goods tend to stick to the pan more. Another way to cut the fat in baked goods is to use two egg whites and one yolk when a recipe calls for two whole eggs. You can also substitute low-fat or skimmed milk for whole milk.

Breakfast – The Hardest Meal to Change

Most people adjust quickly to a high-fibre, low-fat diet, but let me offer a few breakfast suggestions to get you started. For breakfast, bacon and sausage with toast smothered in butter and marmalade are out. Eggs should be limited to two to three a week. Eat more high-fibre cereals. Substitute whole fruits for fruit juices. When I do have eggs, I make them into a nice big omelette, with cottage cheese, onion and tomato. I have wholemeal toast without butter, but sometimes use a low-calorie jam.

I have got into the habit of eating my low-fat dinner left-overs for breakfast by chopping them up with vegetables and cooking them in a nonstick pan with a little chicken stock. Another breakfast idea is grilled fish with potato pancakes made with skimmed milk and browned in a nonstick pan. I'll even have an occasional steak (21 per cent fat) for breakfast.

Restaurant Eating

I am an extensive traveller, so my downfall has been eating out. For most people dining out is a treat, and they can afford to splurge on their calories once in a while. But when you have to eat many meals a week out, you'd better learn some tricks.

First of all, beware of the 'dieter's special' – sirloin steak, cottage cheese and tomato slices. That clever little ploy makes you think you're eating a low-calorie dinner, but it adds up to 730 calories and 70 per cent fat!

Which Foods Are the Fattiest?

It's easy to calculate*:

$$100 \times \left(\frac{\text{grams of fat} \times 9}{\text{total calories}} \right) = \%\text{ calories from fat}$$

Examples:

1 tin tuna in oil = 177 calories
8 grams fat
about 3 oz (75 g) serving

$$100 \times \left(\frac{8 \times 9}{177} \right) = 41\%\text{ fat}$$

1 tin tuna in brine = 120 calories
1.5 grams fat
about 3 oz (75 g) serving

$$100 \times \left(\frac{1.5 \times 9}{120} \right) = 11\%\text{ fat}$$

2% low-fat milk is really 36% fat calories!

8 fl oz (250 ml) = 125 calories
5 grams fat

$$100 \times \left(\frac{5 \times 9}{125} \right) = 36\%\text{ fat}$$

*Calories and grams of fat per serving are listed on most food labels.

When entering a restaurant, I usually ask the waitress to bring me a bowl of the soup of the day and some wholemeal bread right away. Then, while I'm eating that and getting filled up, I decide what I would like to eat *without looking at the menu*. I might decide on fish (which I'll order steamed, poached, or grilled, with lemon juice), or a seafood salad (low calorie dressing, lemon juice, or a dressing mixed with milk), or some kind of bean dish. If I'm with a lady friend, we both have soup and then order just one main dish, which we share. Try to order all your dishes 'dry'; that is, no mayonnaise or butter on the sandwiches, no sauces on the main course, no dressings on the salads. Or ask the waiter to bring these separately so that you can control how much is added to the dish. A little hot milk or mustard moistens a baked potato and makes it very tasty. You can also use milk instead of cream in your coffee. Avoid menu items described as 'dipped in batter', 'fried', 'creamed', or 'in a sauce'. If you order alcoholic drinks, add bottled water, soda water, or a diet mixer to your wine or spirits. Consider stopping at a shop for fresh fruit, low-fat yoghurt, and a wholemeal roll to eat in your hotel room or in a park as a break from restaurants.

One of my co-workers has an interesting restaurant trick. Let's say she orders a turkey sandwich, careful to specify wholemeal bread with no mayonnaise or butter. Everything seems perfect. But her sandwich arrives accompanied by a mound of richly mayonnaised potato salad. Undismayed, she drenches the potato salad with so much salt that no one could possibly eat it. That way she isn't tempted to eat the salad later. The first time I saw her do this, she had ordered a fruit salad and was vigorously launching a salt attack on the sorbet that came with it. Screwy – but effective.

7

Analysing the Diet

Now the Target becomes more complex, but infinitely more useful. Several more concentric rings have been drawn on the target, enabling us to separate the foods more precisely. In the Meat and Milk groups I have arranged the rings so that each new ring of foods contains 5 more grams of fat than those in the preceding ring. I call 5 grams of fat 'one fat' (which is 45 calories), 10 grams of fat 'two fats', etc. The horizontal line across the middle of the circle has numbers printed above and below it. The numbers above the line refer to the number of fats contained in the foods in that segment of the ring; the numbers below the line refer to the number of fibre units contained in the foods in that segment of the ring.

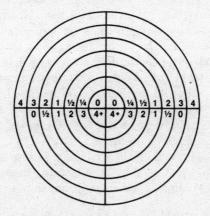

Don't be put off by the figures that follow. If it's easier for you, round off the fractions, as I do. Your results will be close enough. Just keep these basics in mind for each food.

Nutritious Calories

1 meat serving	= 110 calories
1 milk serving	= 80 calories
1 fruit and vegetable serving	= 40 calories
1 bread and cereal serving	= 70 calories

Exceptions:

* The food contains 100 extra carbohydrate calories.

** The food contains 40 fewer carbohydrate calories.

Empty Calories

1 fat	= 45 calories
1 sugar	= 45 calories
1 alcohol	= 105 calories

Now, looking at the large Target on pages 62–63, notice that $3\frac{1}{2}$ oz (100 g) of lean ham in the Meat Group have two fats. Note that $3\frac{1}{2}$ oz (100 g) of veal escalope have three fats. Since every gram of fat contains 9 calories, the two fats in ham contribute 90 calories to the ham. However, there are also 110 calories of protein in the ham, yielding a total of 200 calories for the $3\frac{1}{2}$ oz (100 g). Note that this also allows you to estimate the percentage of fat in the ham: 90 calories of fat out of a total of 200 calories means that the serving is about 45 per cent fat. Conceptually, we are dividing the ham into two parts – the nutritious protein/iron/niacin part equalling 110 calories and the fat part containing 90 calories.

Similarly, the veal escalope contains nutritious protein/iron/niacin equalling 110 calories and three fats contributing 135 calories. Although the nutritious part of the ham and the veal escalope is the same, the fat is higher in the escalope, so it's lower in nutrient density.

You might ask why I pick 3½ oz (100 g) of meat rather than 3 or 5 oz (75 or 150 g) or some other number. In fact, how come all the foods on the Target are shown in precise quantities? The reason is that I wanted the portion size to reflect a logical serving size – something that people are used to – and to contain a specified calorie value for the nutritious part of the food. In other words, I picked the portion size of each food on the chart very carefully. I wanted the portion (or serving size) to supply the vitamins and minerals considered typical of a serving in the respective food group. Any food you select from the Meat Group has a protein/vitamin/mineral content similar to that of any other selection in the Meat Group, and each selection will supply approximately 110 calories *before* you add the number of fats it contains.

The serving sizes I have chosen are usually the same as those that dietitians have used for years in menu planning. A later chapter gives details on how to remember these serving sizes.

If we select a food like 2½ oz (65 g) of cooked brown rice in the second ring below the horizontal line across the middle of the Target, we can assume that it contains the vitamins and minerals expected of a serving in the Bread and Cereal Group. We also know that it contains 70 calories, because each serving of bread and cereal contains 70 calories. And we know from the number 1 printed just below the horizontal line in that segment of the Target that it contains one unit of fibre. Similarly, one slice of bread equals one serving and is assigned a caloric value of 70 calories. (Not all slices of bread contain exactly 70 calories, but they are close enough to make this system useful.)

Doughnuts are near the periphery of the Bread and Cereal Group. One doughnut gives zero fibre as you can see from the 0 printed below the horizontal line in that segment. A doughnut also contains one fat and a half sugar. In the same way that one fat means 5 grams of fat, one sugar means 11.5 grams of sugar, or 45 calories. Thus it becomes easy to count fats and sugars, since one of either equals 45 calories. If I eat a doughnut, I know that it contains:

1 fat × 45 calories	=	45 calories of fat
½ sugar × 45 calories	=	22 calories of sugar
Nutritious material (protein, carbohydrate)	=	70 calories
		137 calories

The best way to make the Target a useful tool in your own day-to-day diet is to analyse some hypothetical menus. I'll analyse some good and some not-so-good ways to eat. If you'll take the time to go through this with me, you'll learn how to analyse your own eating patterns.

The list of foods below might represent the food intake for one day for a male vegetarian. Let's analyse it to see if he is a smart vegetarian.

Breakfast

1 oz (25 g) muesli
4 fl oz (120 ml) low-fat milk
4 fl oz (120 ml) grapefruit juice

1 cup coffee
1 teaspoon top of the milk

Lunch

Grilled-cheese sandwich containing:
1⅓ oz (35 g) mild Cheddar
2 slices wholemeal bread
1 teaspoon mayonnaise

½ teaspoon butter
3 oz (75 g) dried apricots
1 natural fruit juice soft drink – 12 fl oz (350 ml)

Snack
1½ oz (40 g) sunflower seeds

Dinner
Salad containing:

about 8 oz (225 g) lettuce and assorted vegetables	4 oz (115 g) full fat cottage cheese
2 tablespoons Italian dressing	1 slice French bread
4 fl oz (120 ml) carrot juice	1 teaspoon butter
	4 oz (115 g) ice cream

Our vegetarian started the day with 1 oz (25 g) muesli and 4 fl oz (120 ml) low-fat milk. Let's assume that the muesli was one of the early commercial varieties that was high in sugar and fat. You will find muesli in the second ring of the Bread and Cereal Group. A 1 oz (25 g) portion of muesli is shown as one serving and it contains one fibre plus one fat and a half sugar. Turn to the 'Dumb Vegetarian' Food Analysis sheet at the end of the chapter, where you will see that you should put a 1 in the Bread and Cereal column, a 1 in the Fibre column, a 1 in the Fat column, and a ½ in the Sugar column. The 4 fl oz (120 ml) of low-fat milk gets a ½ in the Milk column and a ½ in the Fat column. The 4 fl oz (120 ml) of grapefruit juice is in the third ring on the Target and rates a 1 in the Fruit and Vegetable column, a ½ in the Fibre column, and a ½ in the Sugar column. The cup of coffee doesn't warrant a mark in any column. The teaspoon of top of the milk he used is mostly fat and has to be assigned a value. Top of the milk doesn't appear on the Target. Extras that are added to foods but aren't really foods themselves can be found in a special list on page 132. From this list you find that 1 teaspoon top of the milk receives a ⅓ mark in the Fat column and nothing else. I don't put such 'nonfoods' on the

Target. Substances that are almost pure fat or pure sugar will be found on the Extras list.

A grilled-cheese sandwich and a soft drink were on the lunch menu. Mild Cheddar is in the third ring of the Milk Group, and $1\frac{1}{3}$ oz (35 g) are considered one serving. The cheese gets a 1 in the Milk column and a 2 in the Fat column. Note that 40 calories must be *substracted* from the usual number of calories given by the Milk-Group servings. A double asterisk (**) next to a food indicates that it has 40 fewer carbohydrate calories. Put it on the analysis sheet, and I'll show you how to handle it later. That much cheese, in other words, contains 10 grams of fat, which I call two fats. Two slices of wholemeal bread get a 2 in the Bread and Cereal column and, because they were wholemeal, a 4 in the Fibre column. Mayonnaise isn't really a food so it's on the Extras list. One teaspoon gets a 1 in the Fat column. Butter, also a nonfood, deserves to be recorded in the Fat column only. Dried apricots are quite high in sugar, so they are in the second ring of the Fruit and Vegetable Group. A 3 oz (75 g) portion yields a 1 in the Fruit and Vegetable column and a 2 in the Fibre column. Note that it also contains two sugars. The soft drink may be 'natural', but as it contains only sugar, it's a nonfood on the Extras list. It supplies three sugars.

The sunflower seeds are likely to fool you. They go in the Meat Group all right, but way out on the periphery because they are so high in fat. I'm afraid that a lot of vegetarians and health food buffs think of seeds as rich sources of protein. They are rich sources of fat with a little protein added. Our imaginary vegetarian ate $1\frac{1}{2}$ oz (40 g) of sunflower seeds, and the Target shows 3 oz (75 g) as one serving, so enter a $\frac{1}{2}$ in the Meat column, about $2\frac{3}{4}$ in the Fat column, and a $\frac{3}{4}$ in the Fibre column.

At this point, I'm sure you can see the logic and practicality of the Target, so I will discuss the other foods quickly. The 8 oz (225 g) lettuce and assorted vegetables earn a 2 in the Fruit and Vegetable column and a 4 in the Fibre column. Salad dressing is only fat. Carrot juice receives marks in three columns on the analysis sheet. Be careful with the cottage cheese. It appears twice in the Milk Group on the Target because one can get low-fat or sometimes full fat cottage cheese. Our vegetarian picked the wrong kind and gets a 1 in the Fat column in addition to the 1 in the Milk column. French bread and butter you can do easily enough by yourself. The ice cream is a little tricky. A serving of ice cream, according to the Target, is 8 oz (225 g) but our vegetarian had only 4 oz (115 g), or approximately one-half a serving. So we have to give him half the marks of a full serving; that is, only a 2 in the Fat column instead of a 4, a $\frac{1}{2}$ in the Milk column, and about $1\frac{1}{3}$ in the Sugar column.

Now we can do an analysis of the day's food; I imagine you will be surprised at the amount of information we are able to obtain. To organise this information, add up the marks in each column. As you look at the totals, it should leap out at you that our subject hasn't eaten a balanced diet. He got only half a serving in the Meat Group, which means he will be short on iron and niacin for that day. If our vegetarian were a woman, the low iron intake would be twice as significant because women need twice as much iron as men. Typically, when people's Meat-Group choices are low for the day, one finds them high in the milks and/or breads, which supply plenty of protein. Our vegetarian followed this pattern, so we don't have to be as concerned about his protein intake as we are about his iron and niacin requirements. He exceeded the minimum two servings in the Milk Group and the minimum four servings in both the Fruit and Vegetable Group and the Bread and Cereal Group.

You should begin your analysis by looking at the first

four columns and judging the nutrient intake for the day. Keep in mind the leader nutrients of each food group (see page 11). If, for example, a person eats fewer than four servings of fruits and vegetables, you should immediately suspect a low vitamin A or vitamin C intake. Fewer than two servings in the Milk Group may indicate insufficient calcium and riboflavin.

Next, calculate the *number of calories* from each column. Our vegetarian had a total of half a serving in the Meat column, and each serving contains 110 calories, so he got 55 'nutritious' calories from meats. Three servings of milk yield 240 calories, but don't forget to subtract the 40 calories that we noted earlier. When you add up the food group nutritious calories, the total comes to 735.

Now, add up the marks in the other columns and multiply by the calories shown. For example, sixteen fats at 45 calories each yield 720 calories. Fibre, in our system, is noncaloric. Eight sugars yield 360 calories. Our vegetarian had no alcohol, so the total of 'empty' calories is 1080. More than half his calories for the day came from fat and sugar (supplying him with no nutrition at all) and, despite being a vegetarian, he got fewer than the fifteen minimum daily fibres I recommend. He expects to get all the vitamins/minerals/protein he needs for the day from only 735 calories of real food. He is probably the kind of person who gets ill all the time and takes vitamin supplements because 'our foods are grown in depleted soil'. The truth is that his own poor food selections are responsible for any nutritional deficiency. I call him our dumb vegetarian; in the next chapter you will see that it is quite possible to be a smart vegetarian.

Dumb Vegetarian Food Analysis

Instructions on page 61

Quantity	Food	Meat	Milk	Fruit & Vegetable	Bread & Cereal	Fibre	Fat	Sugar	Alcohol
				Servings				Target Units	
1 oz (25 g)	Muesli		½		1	1	1	½	
4 fl oz (120 ml)	Low-fat milk						½	½	
4 fl oz (120 ml)	Grapefruit juice			1		½			
1 cup	Coffee								
1 tsp.	Top of the milk		1 (—40)				⅓		
1½ oz (35 g)	Mild Cheddar						2		
2 slices	Wholemeal bread				2	4			
1 tsp.	Mayonnaise						1		
½ tsp.	Butter						½		
3 oz (75 g)	Dried apricots			1		2		2	
12 fl oz (350 ml)	Natural soft drink							3	
1½ oz (40g)	Sunflower seeds	½				¾	2¾		
8 oz (225 g)	Lettuce/vegetables			2		4			
2 tbsp.	Salad dressing						4		
4 fl oz (120 ml)	Carrot juice			1		½			
4 oz (115 g)	Cottage cheese		1				1	½	
1 slice	French bread				1	½			
1 tsp.	Butter						1		
4 oz (115 g)	Ice cream		½				2	1⅓	
Totals:		½	3	5	4	13	16	8	0
		×110	×80	×40	×70		×45	×45	×105
		55	240 −40 200	200	280		720	360	0

Empty Calories 1080

Total Calories 1815 = 60% Empty Calories

Fat Calories 720

Total Calories 1815 = 40% Fat Calories

Total Nutritious Calories = 735

Total Empty Calories = 1080

8

The Smart Vegetarian

Again using the Target, let's analyse the following vegetarian menu plan.

Breakfast
2 biscuits Shredded Wheat with 8 fl oz (250 ml) skimmed milk

¼ pint (150 ml) plain yoghurt
½ grapefruit

Lunch
1 apricot
¾ pint (450 ml) split-pea soup

1 slice pumpernickel bread

Snack
2½ oz (65 g) carrot/celery sticks

2 oz (50 g) dip made of low-fat cottage cheese and dry onion soup mix

Dinner
3 bean tortillas made of
  9 oz (275 g) pinto beans
  6 oz (175 g) low-fat cottage cheese
  Pickles
  3 wholemeal tortillas

Tossed salad made of
  8 oz (225 g) lettuce/vegetables
  2 tablespoons non-oil salad dressing
6 oz (175 g) fresh sliced strawberries

Two Shredded Wheat biscuits rate a 2 mark in the Bread and Cereal column and an 8 in the Fibre column. Be careful with the milk used in the cereal! Milk is listed three times on the Target, but the menu calls for skimmed milk, which is in the bull's-eye. The ¼ pint (150 ml) plain yoghurt, also in the bull's-eye, earns a 1 in the Milk column and no marks in the Fat column. Since grapefruit is a large fruit, half of one grapefruit equals one serving in the Fruit and Vegetable column and gets a 2 in the Fibre column.

It's awfully easy to be lazy when reading a book like this, letting the author do all the thinking for you. Please take the time to locate each food in the menu on the Target and make sure that the analysis sheet is correct. In fact, I have deliberately analysed one of the foods incorrectly. See if you can find it.

Be careful with the split-pea soup! It takes 8 fl oz (250 ml) soup to equal a serving in the Meat Group. Note also that for each serving you have to add 100 additional calories in the Meat column – not in the Fat column. An asterisk (*) next to a food indicates that it has 100 extra calories. The non-oil salad dressing doesn't get marks in any column.

Have you found the mistake yet? Strawberries deserve a 2 in the Fibre column. Change it on the analysis sheet, and then the fibres total a spectacular 44½ for the day – much more in keeping with the fibre intake that I would like to see.

When you total up the columns, the Meat Group has 3½ servings times 110 calories each, but you have to add the extra 350 calories from the complex carbohydrates provided by the peas and beans. The Meat Group gives a total of 735 nutritious calories. Total the four nutrition columns for 1695 calories for the day. Total the fat, sugar and alcohol columns at only 90 calories.

The day's menu provides the minimum acceptable number of servings in each food group plus plenty of fibre,

Smart Vegetarian Food Analysis

Instructions on page 61

Quantity	Food	Meat	Milk	Fruit & Vegetable	Bread & Cereal	Fibre	Fat	Sugar	Alcohol
2 bisc.	Shredded Wheat				2	8			
8 fl oz (250 ml)	Skimmed milk		1						
½	Grapefruit			1		2			
	Apricot			1		2			
¼ pint (150 ml)	Plain yoghurt		1						
¾ pint (450 ml)	Split-pea soup	2 (+200)			1	2	10		
1 slice	Pumpernickel bread					1		½	
2½ oz (65 g)	Carrots/celery			½					
2 oz (50 g)	Low-fat Cottage cheese		½				¼		
9 oz (275 g)	Pinto beans	1½ (+150)				7½	⅜		
6 oz (175 g)	Cottage cheese		1½				¾		
3	Wholemeal tortillas				3	6			
8 oz (225 g)	Lettuce/vegetables			2		4			
6 oz (175 g)	Strawberries			1		1			
	Totals:	3½	4	5½	6	43½	2	0	0
		×110	×80	×40	×70		×45	×45	×105
		385	320	220	420		90		0
		+ 350					90		
		735							

Servings — Meat, Milk, Fruit & Vegetable, Bread & Cereal

Target Units — Fat, Sugar, Alcohol

Total Nutritious Calories = 1695   Total Empty Calories = 90

Empty Calories   90
Total Calories   1785   = 5% Empty Calories

Fat Calories   90
Total Calories 1785   = 5% Fat Calories

all from just 1695 calories because only 90 of the calories (approximately 5 per cent) came from sugar and fat and alcohol. If you compare this with the analysis in the previous chapter, you will see that our smart vegetarian had not only a greater quantity of food but also a much higher nutrient density for the same number of calories. He did this partly by lowering the sugar content of the food but mostly by lowering the fat content. As I have pointed out repeatedly, it's fat in the diet that dramatically raises the calories while decreasing the nutrient density. Unfortunately, many of the foods formerly considered nutritious, such as the meats, whole-milk products, and nuts, are the worst offenders. Those who favour dairy products are lucky because we can use skimmed-milk products. The beef eaters may not be so lucky – it's hard to buy a skimmed steak.

9

What's a Serving?

From your reading of the previous chapters, it should be obvious that 'servings' and 'serving size' are integral to the Target method of analysing diets. I urge my readers, particularly my male readers, not to skip over the following discussion.

If you are like me, you don't want to think about fiddly measures or what someone else says is a serving. For us, a serving has meant whatever we put on our plates. The 'little woman' gets a little serving and the 'man of the house' gets a big serving. Keep thinking that way, and you will soon become a fat 'man of the house'.

Nutritionists (and cooks) have confused us long enough. It's time to put numbers on food. It isn't all that hard! If the average man makes a cup out of his hands, as if he were trying to get a scoop of water out of a stream, his hands will hold about 8 fl oz (250 ml). Obviously, if you have huge paws it won't work. Remember, also, that it takes 3 teaspoons to equal 1 tablespoon. You get $3\frac{1}{2}$ oz (100 g) of meat in a McDonald's Big Mac. Remember these three clues and read this chapter with care.

Two, two, four and four is the quick way to remember how many servings you should eat each day from the four food groups. These numbers change a bit for a pregnant woman or a fast-growing teenager, but I don't want to confuse the issue, so let's assume for now that you are an average, nonpregnant adult. You need two servings from the Meat Group, two servings from the Milk Group, four servings from the Fruit and Vegetable Group, and four servings from the Bread and Cereal Group. These are minimum requirements – if you eat no more than this each day you will just barely squeak by in your daily vitamin and mineral requirements. Eating more than the minimum serving requirements will make you nutritionally safer but might add too many unwanted calories if you're overfat and need to lose weight. If you're one of these people, careful selection from the centre of the Target is a must!

Let me go through each food group, describing the serving sizes that are used in the dietary analyses.

Two from the Meat Group

The standard serving size in the Meat Group is $3\frac{1}{2}$ oz (100 g), the same as in a Big Mac hamburger (it's 4 oz (115 g) before cooking but shrinks to $3\frac{1}{2}$ oz (100 g)). In other words, a 12 oz (350 g) steak is much more than a serving from the point of view of nutritional analysis. In fact, it is considered to be approximately three and a half servings in the Meat Group.

So any time you eat a pork chop or a steak, just form a mental picture of a Big Mac and judge accordingly how many servings you are getting. Fish is lower in fat than beef but also a little lower in vitamins and minerals. Consequently, you can eat a little more – $4\frac{1}{2}$ oz (130 g) – to equal $3\frac{1}{2}$ oz (100 g) of beef nutritionally. This is great for dieters who want more quantity without more calories.

When you move into the non-animal meats – nuts, seeds, beans and legumes – you have to eat about twice as much in order to get the comparable amounts of vitamins and minerals found in beef. For beans and legumes this is a good deal. I like being able to double the quantity of food I eat without doubling the calories. Since there is practically no fat in the beans and legumes you can eat 8 oz (225 g) cooked and get no more calories than if you ate only 3½ oz (100 g) of hamburger. This is because the beans are only 4½ per cent fat while the hamburger is 60 per cent fat. When you eat nuts and seeds, the deal isn't as good. To get the comparable nutrition of a 3½ oz (100 g) piece of beef, you need to eat about 3½ oz (100 g) of nuts, which adds up to 585 calories because the fat is up to 85 per cent!

Two from the Milk Group

In the Milk Group the standard serving size is 8 fl oz (250 ml) of milk. This is true whether you have whole milk, skimmed milk, chocolate milk or buttermilk. The calories differ because of the varying fat or sugar content, but the vitamin and mineral content is nearly the same in all these liquids. When you eat yoghurt, the liquid content is slightly less, so that ¼ pint (150 ml) becomes the serving size. In other words, the vitamins and minerals in ¼ pint (150 ml) yoghurt are about equal to the vitamins and minerals in 8 fl oz (250 ml) of milk. When you eat cottage cheese, even more water is eliminated, and only 4 oz (115 g) is needed to be nutritionally equal to a whole cup of milk. When you eat ice cream a serving size is a good 8 oz (250 g). Whoopee! Do you know why you can eat more? You have to eat that much ice cream in order to get the same amount of vitamins and minerals that you get in 8 fl oz (250 ml) milk! 8 fl oz (250 ml) skimmed milk with only 80 calories has the same nutritional value as 8 oz (225 g) of ice cream at 400 calories.

The standard serving size for the hard cheeses is 1⅓ oz (35 g). This is easy to remember if you picture in your mind one of those pre-wrapped slices of cheese that you put on a cheeseburger. They are usually sold as eight individual slices to an 8-oz (225 g) package. So one of these slices plus a third of another is one serving in the Milk Group and equals the vitamins and minerals in 8 fl oz (250 ml) of milk. I always get a laugh out of the men in my audiences who claim they never eat anything from the Milk Group. Later at a cocktail party, I see them eating handfuls of the 1 inch (2.5 cm) cubes of cheese from the hors d'oeuvre tray. If you folded up 1⅓ slices of the pre-wrapped cheese it would form a 1-inch (2.5 cm) cube. You could practically inhale it without a second thought! While one of those innocent-looking little cubes may have the same vitamin and mineral content as a glass of skimmed milk, it has double the calories because of the fat it contains.

Again, I appeal to you not to skip through this material carelessly. Just think of 8 fl oz (250 ml) of fluid milk as a serving and then decrease the serving size in your mind as the milk products get 'drier'. Squeeze a little water out of the 8 fl oz (250 ml) milk and you have yoghurt – ¼ pint (150 ml) equals a serving. Squeeze almost all the water out and you have hard cheese – a 1-inch (2.5 cm) cube equals a serving.

Four from the Fruit and Vegetable Group

In the fruits and vegetables the standard serving size is about 4 oz (125 g). Generally, this is one whole fruit or vegetable; that is, a whole apple, a whole pear, one carrot, one potato, etc. If the fruit or vegetable is large (grapefruit, Charentais melon, aubergine), then only half of it constitutes a serving.

When you dry or extract the juice from a fruit or liquidise a vegetable, the serving size is 4 fl oz (115 ml). For example, 6 oz (175 g) plums has the same vitamin content as 3 oz (75 g) prunes (dried plums) or 4 fl oz (120 ml) prune juice. But remember – the sugar content increases dramatically in the dried fruit or fruit juice.

Four from the Bread and Cereal Group

In the breads and cereals we separate the solid products (such as breads, buns, cakes) from the loose products (such as barley, rice, cereals). For the solid products the standard serving size is 1 slice of bread. Hamburger buns, hot dog buns, baps and so on, all equal 2 slices of bread.

For the loose grain products the standard serving size is 1 oz (25 g) of the cooked or prepared food and that has about the same nutritional value as 1 slice of bread.

Others

When you eat a casserole type of dish or a combination of foods prepared in a restaurant, break down the dish into its individual components and then analyse it.

Examples

1 serving lasagna contains

1 serving pasta (Bread and Cereal Group)
½ serving vegetable
2 servings cheese
½ serving meat

1 vegetarian omelette contains

3 eggs
1 oz (25 g) cheese
½ oz (15 g) butter
1 serving vegetable

10

The All-American Diet

If we now proceed to analyse more complicated menus, diets and recipes, we find that there isn't enough room on the Target to print the names of all the foods. In my office I have a huge Target that covers an entire wall behind my desk, but it's a little difficult to carry around with me, and it wouldn't fit into this book. So I have taken all the foods on my big Target and printed them in tables, which you will find in the Appendix. If you can't find a food on the Target, you can find it in the tables if you look in the proper food group.

Let's analyse another day's menu, this time using the tables to supplement the Target. The menu printed on the following page is supposed to represent the food intake of a typical American for one day. I call it the All-American Diet.

You can tell at a glance that our all-American eats a high-fat diet, but the analysis will point out just how incredibly fat it is. Look up eggs on the Target, and you find that two eggs equal one serving in the Meat Group and contain two fats. Now flip to the Appendix and look for eggs in the Meat Group (listed under Miscellaneous). The table gives the same information as the Target, listing two eggs as one meat serving containing two fats, no sugar and no alcohol. Don't overlook the double asterisk that appears next to the eggs both on the Target and in the tables. This sign means subtract 40 calories from the usual

110 calories expected from a serving of meat.

One teaspoon of butter, being almost pure grease, is found only on our Extras list and deserves a 1 in the Fat column.

Breakfast

2 eggs fried in
   1 teaspoon butter
3 rashers bacon
3 pancakes with
   2 teaspoons butter and
   2 tablespoons syrup

4 fl oz (120 ml) orange juice
1 cup of coffee with
   1 teaspoon sugar and
   1 tablespoon top of the milk

Lunch

Cheeseburger made with
   1 hamburger bun
   3½ oz (100 g) minced beef
   2 slices tomato
   1 slice onion
   Lettuce
   1⅓ oz (35 g) mild Cheddar
   1 teaspoon mayonnaise

French fries (about 6 oz) (175 g)
Chocolate shake made with
   8 fl oz (250 ml) whole milk
   8 oz (225 g) vanilla ice cream
   2 tablespoons chocolate syrup

Dinner

4 slices cheese and pepperoni pizza
10 oz (300 g) tossed salad with

4 tablespoons Roquefort dressing
2 lagers

Movies

4 oz (115 g) popcorn with
   1 oz (25 g) butter

1 Coke (12 fl oz (350 ml))
1 choc ice

Bacon can be found on the Target, which indicates that 6 rashers constitute one meat serving and get 3 fat marks. In the table, the same amount of bacon gets 3½ fat marks. When you come across a small discrepancy like this, always rely on the tables for greater accuracy. Because space was limited, it was necessary to round off some numbers on the Target. If 6 rashers constitute a serving and our subject ate only 3, he ate half a serving in the Meat Group and got about $1\frac{3}{4}$ in the Fat column. Don't forget to subtract 20 calories for the double asterisk.

Our all-American also had three pancakes, which you will find in the Bread and Cereal section. One pancake, comparable to a slice of bread in size, is one bread and cereal serving, one-half fat, and one-half fibre. As I have pointed out before, one can make pancakes at home with much less fat, but I am going to assume that these are typical restaurant pancakes. So, three pancakes warrant a 3 in the Bread and Cereal column, a $1\frac{1}{2}$ in the Fibre column, and a $1\frac{1}{2}$ in the Fat column. Butter and syrup are on the Extras list. Orange juice is located in the Fruits and Vegetables, while sugar and top of the milk are on the Extras list.

Notice the way the marks in the Fat column are increasing while marks in the nutrition columns are pretty sparse! Each fat mark equals 45 calories of vitamin/mineral-free grease. That's the way fat in the diet sneaks up on us.

Please work your way through the rest of the analysis by yourself. Once again I have deliberately put an error on the analysis sheet. Can you find it? From here on, I will deal only with those foods on the menu that might present a problem.

In analysing a diet, you will often find you don't know the exact amount of food eaten so you'll just have to make a rough guess. I did this with the tomato, onion and lettuce on the hamburger. I reckoned that they would add up to about $2\frac{1}{2}$ oz (65 g) which equals a $\frac{1}{2}$ mark in the Fruit and Vegetable column and a 1 mark in the Fibre column. In the evening our all-American had a tossed salad, and this time

I knew how much he ate but not exactly which kinds of vegetables. So I just used the old rule of thumb again: 10 oz (300 g) vegetables equals a 1 mark in the Fruit and Vegetable column and a 2 mark in the Fibre column.

French fries are found under Combination Foods, Fast Foods and Soups, as are the pizza and popcorn. Popcorn, you'll notice, earns calories and fibre, but no marks in the nutrition columns.

Did the Roquefort dressing fool you? It stacks up to a 10 mark in the Fat column. The choc ice was another food to guess at. I reckoned that it was about half a serving of ice cream covered with about 2 tablespoons of chocolate.

Did you find the mistake? I gave the french fries only a 3 mark in the Fat column instead of a 4.

We can now total all the columns; the first thing to notice is that all the nutrition columns have more than adequate marks. That is, our subject is not short in any of the four food groups, meaning that his vitamin/mineral/protein requirements are well met – even exceeded. This is typical in the West, where rich food is the norm. Youngsters and most men typically eat a lot, so they are rarely deficient in nutrients. This helps to explain my statement that most people do not need to take vitamin/mineral pills because most people eat high-vitamin/mineral – high-fat foods. The price they pay is obesity. Once they become obese, people cut down on calorie intake, which leads to borderline vitamin/mineral intake.

One cannot have a low-calorie nutritious diet that is high in fat.

One can *have a* high-*calorie nutritious diet that is high in fat.*

When we correct for my deliberate error with the french fries, we calculate that our subject ate 1535 nutritious calories from the four food groups and 3302 calories that were empty of vitamins and protein. It's a fun diet, it's fast food, but it's not smart.

All-American Diet Analysis Sheet

Quantity	Food	Meat	Milk	Fruit & Vegetable	Bread & Cereal	Fibre	Fat	Sugar	Alcohol
2	Eggs	1 (−40)					2		
1 tsp.	Butter						1		
3 rashers	Bacon	½ (−20)					1¾		
3	Pancakes				3		1½		
2 tsp.	Butter						2		
3 tbsp.	Syrup							3	
4 fl oz (120 ml)	Orange juice			1		1½			
1 tsp.	Sugar							½	
1 tbsp.	Top of the milk						1	⅓	
	Hamburger bun				2	½			
3½ oz (100 g)	Minced beef	1					3½		
2⅓ oz (65 g)	American cheese		1 (−40)	½			2⅓		
1⅓ oz (35 g)	Assorted vegetables					1			
1 tsp.	Mayonnaise						1		
6 oz (175 g)	French fries			1		1	3		
8 fl oz (250 ml)	Whole milk		1				1⅔		
8 oz (225 g)	Ice cream		1			½	4⅓	2½	
2 tbsp.	Chocolate syrup							2	
4 slices	Cheese and pepperoni pizza				4	2	8		
2	Lagers	1	4 (−160)						2
10 oz (300 g)	Tossed salad			2		4			
5 tbsp.	Salad dressing						10		
4 oz (115 g)	Popcorn (plus 100 calories)					2			
6 tsp.	Butter						6		
1	Coke		½					3	
1	Choc ice						2	1¼	
	Totals:	3½	7½	4½	9	12½	51	13½	2
		×110	×80	×40	×70		×45	×45	×105
		385	600	180	630		2295	607.5	210
		−60	−200						
		325	400						

+ 100 popcorn

Empty Calories 3257

$\dfrac{\text{Total Calories } 4792}{\text{?}}$ = 68% Empty Calories

$\dfrac{\text{Fat Calories } 2295}{\text{Total Calories } 4792}$ = 48% Fat Calories

Total Nutritious Calories = 1535   Total Empty Calories = 3257

How to Use the Target

1. Meats and milks shown on the Target (above the horizontal line) are graded by their fat content. The numbers just above the horizontal line indicate the amount of fat in the foods for that quarter circle. One 'fat' equals 5 grams of fat equals 45 calories.

2. The non-animal products shown on the lower half of the Target are graded by their fibre content, indicated by the numbers just below the horizontal line. Chapter 16 tells how fibre is measured. Try to get a minimum of 15 'fibres' a day.

3. For most adults, the easiest way to get a balanced diet containing all the vitamins, minerals and protein you need is to be sure that each day you eat:

   2 servings from the Meat Group
   2 servings from the Milk Group
   4 servings from the Bread and Cereal Group
   4 servings from the Fruit and Vegetable Group

4. The foods on the Target are shown in quantities that I consider standard serving sizes. For example, one serving of any of the meats shown (3½ oz (100 g) red meat, 7 oz (200 g) legumes, 3 oz (75 g) nuts) will yield almost identical amounts of the protein, vitamins and minerals expected of Meat-Group foods, but, as indicated by the numbers above the horizontal line, quite different amounts of fat.

5. In other words, a serving (as shown) from any good group contains roughly the same number of nutrients as a serving of any other food in the same food group. But the amount of fibre and the amount of non-nutritive sugar and fat can differ greatly.

THE TARGET CONCEPT
Instructions page 61

* = add 100 calories
** = subtract 40 calories

MEATS
1 serving = 110 calories

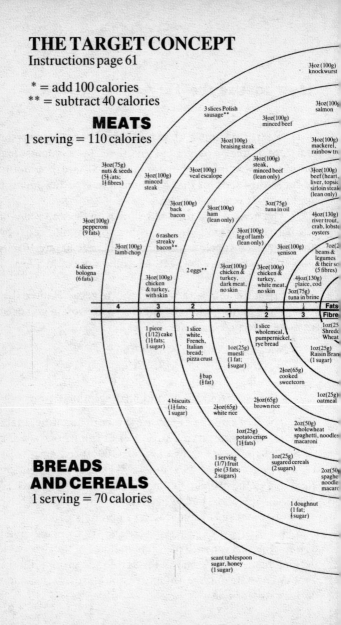

3½oz (100g)
knockwurst

3½oz(100g)
salmon

3 slices Polish
sausage**

3½oz(100g)
minced beef

3½oz(100g)
braising steak

3½oz(100g)
mackerel,
rainbow trout

3½oz(100g)
steak,
minced beef
(lean only)

3½oz(100g)
beef (heart,
liver, topside,
sirloin steak
(lean only)

3½oz(75g)
nuts & seeds
(5½ fats;
1½ fibres)

3½oz(100g)
minced
steak

3½oz(100g)
veal escalope

3oz(75g)
tuna in oil

3½oz(100g)
back
bacon

3½oz(100g)
ham
(lean only)

4½oz(130g)
river trout,
crab, lobster,
oysters

3½oz(100g)
pepperoni
(9 fats)

6 rashers
streaky
bacon**

3½oz(100g)
leg of lamb
(lean only)

7oz(2
beans &
legumes
& their so
(5 fibres)

3½oz(100g)
lamb chop

3½oz(100g)
venison

4 slices
bologna
(6 fats)

2 eggs**

3½oz(100g)
chicken &
turkey,
dark meat,
no skin

3½oz(100g)
chicken &
turkey,
white meat,
no skin

4½oz(130g)
plaice, cod

3oz(75g)
tuna in brine

3½oz(100g)
chicken
& turkey,
with skin

4	3	2	1	½		Fats
0		1		2	3	Fibre

1 piece
(1/12) cake
(1½ fats;
1 sugar)

1 slice
white,
French,
Italian
bread;
pizza crust

1 slice
wholemeal,
pumpernickel,
rye bread

1oz(25
Shredd
Wheat

1oz(25g)
muesli
(1 fat;
½ sugar)

1oz(25g)
Raisin Bran
(1 sugar)

½ bap
(½ fat)

2½oz(65g)
cooked
sweetcorn

4 biscuits
(1½ fats;
1 sugar)

2½oz(65g)
white rice

2½oz(65g)
brown rice

1oz(25g)
oatmeal

1oz(25g)
potato crisps
(1½ fats)

2oz(50g)
wholewheat
spaghetti, noodles,
macaroni

1 serving
(1/7) fruit
pie (3 fats;
2 sugars)

1oz(25g)
sugared cereals
(2 sugars)

2oz(50g)
spaghe
noodles
macaron

1 doughnut
(1 fat;
½ sugar)

BREADS
AND CEREALS
1 serving = 70 calories

scant tablespoon
sugar, honey
(1 sugar)

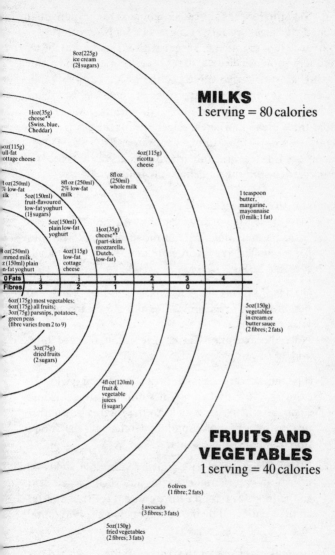

MILKS
1 serving = 80 calories

8oz(225g) ice cream (2½ sugars)

1oz(35g) cheese** (Swiss, blue, Cheddar)

4oz(115g) full-fat cottage cheese

4oz(115g) ricotta cheese

[8fl oz](250ml) 2% low-fat milk

8fl oz (250ml) 2% low-fat milk

8fl oz (250ml) whole milk

5oz(150ml) fruit-flavoured low-fat yoghurt (1½ sugars)

1 teaspoon butter, margarine, mayonnaise (0 milk; 1 fat)

5oz(150ml) plain low-fat yoghurt

1½oz(35g) cheese** (part-skim mozzarella, Dutch, low-fat)

[8oz](250ml) skimmed milk, 5oz (150ml) plain non-fat yoghurt

4oz(115g) low-fat cottage cheese

0 Fats	½	½	1	2	3	4
Fibres	3	2	1	½	0	

6oz(175g) most vegetables; 6oz(175g) all fruits; 3oz(75g) parsnips, potatoes, green peas (fibre varies from 2 to 9)

5oz(150g) vegetables in cream or butter sauce (2 fibres; 2 fats)

3oz(75g) dried fruits (2 sugars)

4fl oz (120ml) fruit & vegetable juices (½ sugar)

FRUITS AND VEGETABLES
1 serving = 40 calories

6 olives (1 fibre; 2 fats)

½ avocado (3 fibres; 3 fats)

5oz(150g) fried vegetables (2 fibres; 3 fats)

6. Sugar in foods is indicated right next to the individual food. One 'sugar' equals 11.5 grams equals 45 calories.

7. Just looking at the Target without using any of its numbers should help you select a better diet. Foods with the highest nutritional value and the fewest calories are in the centre. If you can't resist a piece of apple pie, go ahead, but realise that it is low in fibre and nutrients. Make your other three bread and cereal selections for the day from the centre. Used in this simple qualitative way, the Target becomes a fine teaching tool for youngsters or for those too impatient to study the calculations below.

Analytic Use of the Target

1. (a) One serving of any meat shown yields 110 calories from the nutritious part of the meat plus 45 calories for each 'fat' the meat contains. (One 'fat' equals 5 grams of fat.)

(b) One serving of any milk product yields 80 nutritious calories plus 45 calories for each fat the milk contains.
Note the exceptions in calorie count marked by * and **.

(c) One serving of any bread or cereal yields 70 calories. Note that sometimes non-nutritive fats and sugars are listed right next to the food. The number just below the horizontal line refers to the food's fibre content for that quarter circle.

(d) One serving of any fruit or vegetable yields 40 nutritious calories plus the fats and sugars listed next to the food. The food's fibre content for that quarter circle is indicated by the number below the horizontal line.

2. To make full use of the Target, write down a day's

food intake on one of the analysis sheets in the Appendix. Then analyse each food, using the information on the Target. Each food is divided into its nutritious part and its non-nutritious fats and sugars. List the nutritious part of the food in one of the first four columns (which represent servings) on the analysis sheet. The empty-calorie fat, sugar, and alcohol are listed in the last three columns. Fibre in the food is nutritious but essentially non-caloric and is listed in its own column.

Examples

3. Find 3½ oz (100 g) white-meat chicken with no skin on the Target. It should be entered on the analysis sheet as follows:

> 1 mark in the Meat column because it is one serving of meat. (Each mark in this column yields 110 calories.)
> ½ mark in the Fat column because the number above the horizontal line indicates it contains ½ fat. (Each mark in the Fat column represents 5 grams of fat or 45 calories.)

4. Find 7 oz (200 g) haricot beans on the Target. It should be analysed as follows:

> 1 mark in the Meat column because it is one serving of meat.
> ¼ mark in the Fat column.
> 5 marks in the Fibre column because beans, unlike most meats, contain lots of fibre. Other exceptions to the Target rules are usually noted on the Target right next to the food. (Fibres are explained in Chapter 16.)
> Write '+ 100' next to the mark in the Meat column because the asterisk signifies another exception – a

serving of beans has 100 more calories than the usual 110 calories per meat serving.

5. Find 4 oz (115 g) low-fat cottage cheese on the Target. Analyse it as follows:

> 1 mark in the Milk column (80 calories).
> ½ mark in the Fat column.

> Note that 4 oz (115 g) full-fat cottage cheese warrants 1 mark in the Fat column.

6. Find 1½ oz (35 g) mozzarella cheese on the Target. Analyse it as follows:

> 1 mark in the Milk column.
> 1 mark in the Fat column.
> Write '—40' next to the 1 in the Milk column because the double asterisk means this particular milk product yields 40 fewer calories than the usual 80 calories from the nutritious part of a milk serving. Another exception!

7. Find 6 oz (175 g) fruit on the Target. Analyse it as follows:

> 1 mark in the Fruit and Vegetable column (40 calories).
> 2 marks in the Fibre column.

> If it were 3 oz (175 g) of dried fruit, the analysis would be the same, except for 2 marks in the Sugar column. (1 sugar equals 11.5 grams equals 45 calories.)

8. Find 1 slice wholemeal bread on the Target. Analyse it as follows:

> 1 mark in the Bread and Cereal column (70 calories).
> 2 marks in the Fibre column.

9. Find 1 oz (25 g) muesli on the Target and analyse:

1 mark in the Bread and Cereal column.
1 mark in the Fibre column.
1 mark in the Fat column.
$\frac{1}{2}$ mark in the Sugar column.

How to Use the Tables in the Appendix

If you can't find a food on the Target, look for it in the tables in the Appendix. For example, a food which is almost pure fat or sugar or alcohol is listed in the table called Extras on page 132. All other foods are listed under their respective food groups. The units used have been explained above.

The target itself cannot possibly contain every known food. The tables, which are more complete, represent the Target in tabular form.

11

Covert's Eat-All-You-Want Diet

Let's analyse one more day's menu to be sure that the use of the table is clear. This menu is designed for me, to satisfy my typical male urge to eat a lot of food. It's called Covert's Eat-All-You-Want Diet. I'm not going to go over the items individually this time. Let's see if you can do it by yourself. May I suggest that you use one of the Food Analysis sheets in the Appendix to examine my diet without referring to the analysis that appears on page 71. Once you are done, check yours against mine.

Breakfast

2 Shredded Wheat biscuits mixed with
   1 oz (25 g) Raisin Bran

8 fl oz (250 ml) skimmed milk
½ sliced banana
½ grapefruit

Lunch

8 oz (225 g) vegetarian chilli
2 oz (50 g) whole tomatoes
Tuna sandwich made with
   2 slices wholemeal bread
   3 oz (175 g) tuna in brine
   2 teaspoons low-calorie mayonnaise (half the calories of ordinary)

4 oz (115 g) low fat cottage cheese
8 fl oz (250 ml) chocolate milk (1% fat)

Dinner

2 skinned baked chicken
  breasts
1 baked potato
5 tablespoons yoghurt
  dressing
4 oz (115 g) broccoli with
  lemon juice
2 slices wholemeal bread

8 oz (225 g) tossed salad
2½ tablespoons salad
  dressing made with no
  oil
½ cantaloupe melon
2 glasses wine, diluted with
  water, or about 6 fl oz
  (175 ml) wine

Movies

4 oz (115 g) plain popcorn
1 diet soft drink

Before you start the analysis, scan the menu. You will see
that it supplies a lot of food. The actual quantity probably
equals that of the All-American Diet, yet the Eat-All-You-
Want Diet supplies far more vitamins and minerals and
three times as much fibre. It seems to me that anyone who
eats these foods for a day would not feel deprived.

Notice that the Eat-All-You-Want Diet supplies more
than the minimum two, two, four, and four servings from
the four food groups, so that safe vitamin/mineral/protein
intake is assured. Notice also that the number of servings
from the bottom half of the Target is very high. It's easy to
identify and eat low-fat vegetable products, and they allow
us to increase carbohydrate (fibre) intake dramatically
without increasing calorie intake. The Eat-All-You-Want
menu provides only three and a half fats or 158 fat calories
for the day. If total calories for the day come to 2180, then
158 fat calories divided by 2180 indicates that this is a 7
percent fat diet. The All-American Diet was 48 percent fat.
As dietary fat decreases, we want dietary carbohydrate to
increase. In other words, a low-fat/high-fibre diet could
also be called a high-carbohydrate diet. I wish that more

Eat-All-You-Want Diet Food Analysis

Instructions on page 61

Quantity	Food	Meat	Milk	Fruit & Vegetable	Bread & Cereal	Fibre	Fat	Sugar	Alcohol
		Servings					**Target Units**		
2	Shredded Wheat				2	8			
1 oz (25 g)	Raisin Bran				1	4		1	
8 fl oz (250 ml)	Skimmed milk		1						
½	Sliced banana			1		1			
½	Grapefruit			1		1			
8 oz (225 g)	Chili	1 (+100)		¼		5			
2 oz (50 g)	Tomatoes					½			
2 slices	Wholemeal bread				2	4			
3 oz (75 g)	Tuna in brine	1							
2 tsp	Low-calorie mayonnaise						¼		
4 oz (115 g)	Low fat cottage cheese		1						
8 fl oz (250 ml)	Chocolate milk		1				⅓	1⅓	
2	Chicken breasts	2					½		
1	Potato			2		2	½		
5 tbsp	Yoghurt dressing		½						
4 oz (115 g)	Broccoli			1		3			
2 slices	Wholemeal bread				2	4			
8 oz (225 g)	Tossed salad			1½		3			
½	Cantaloupe melon			2		2			
6 fl oz (175 ml)	Wine								1½
1	Popcorn (plus 100 calories)								
4 oz (115 g)	Diet soft drink							0	
	Totals:	4	3½	8¾	7	39½	3½+	2⅓	1½
		×110	×80	×40	×70		×157.5	×45	×105
		440	280	350	490		157.5	105	157.5
		+100					+100 popcorn		
		540							

Total Nutritious Calories = 1660   Total Empty Calories = 520

$\dfrac{\text{Empty Calories} \quad 520}{\text{Total Calories} \quad 2180}$ = 24% Empty Calories

$\dfrac{\text{Fat Calories} \quad 157.5}{\text{Total Calories} \quad 2180}$ = 7% Fat Calories

runners would eat this way instead of trying to 'carbo-hydrate load' before a race. It's important that carbo-hydrate increases show up in the Fibre column, not in the Sugar column. This is essentially what nutritionists mean when they say that we should eat fewer of the simple carbohydrates (sugars) and more of the complex carbo-hydrates.

12

How to Modify a Recipe

Low-fat/high-fibre eating does not have to be dull. Furthermore, you don't have to throw away your favourite cookbook or abandon your favourite recipes. I even encourage gourmet cooking! The trouble with so-called gourmet cooks is that they judge their cooking only by the final taste and appearance of the food. That's no test of a real cook. Anyone who uses enough butter and sugar can make food taste great. Gourmet cooks of the future will make tasty dishes without fat or sugar. The trick is to modify recipes rather than invent new ones. And the most important modification is to decrease fat.

Fat is insidious! You already know that it can boost the calories in a food tremendously without increasing the quantity of the food. It's virtually invisible in meats and cheese and, as an oil, can easily slither into a salad and disappear. One tablespoon of salad dressing is as fattening as *all* the following foods put together: one-half cucumber, 4 oz (115 g) lettuce, one carrot, one tomato, 2 oz (50 g) beetroot, 2 oz (50 g) beans, and nine mushrooms. Yet that little tablespoon of dressing won't increase the bulk of the salad at all. That's why fat is so bad. It adds lots of calories without adding volume. When you sit down to eat, you don't say, 'I think I want about 1500 calories now.' You don't crave calories – you crave food – its taste, texture and quantity. And you probably stop eating when you feel full. Since fat in food doesn't add much volume, you can inadvertently consume many, many calories before you feel full. When you reduce the fat in foods, you can do more eating and less calorie counting. You will feel better satisfied yet consume fewer calories.

Low-fat/high-fibre foods may fill you up while you're eating them, but the feeling of fullness, known as satiety, doesn't last. Fatty foods do provide long-lasting satiety. A low-fat/high fibre diet is synonymous with a high-carbohydrate diet. Carbohydrates, because they are digested quickly, are emptied from the stomach and upper intestine rather quickly, so that lasting satiety is not typically associated with high-carbohydrate diets. However, high-fibre foods are complex carbohydrates, which are harder to digest and have a higher satiety value than the refined flour and sugar foods that are the principal carbohydrates of many people. However, nothing has the satiety value of fat. That's why I encourage more frequent eating on a low-fat/high-fibre diet. Eat three meals a day along with midmorning, midafternoon, and evening snacks.

It makes me smile when people claim that a high-protein breakfast is necessary to carry them through to lunch. They're kidding themselves when they claim that the protein stays their hunger. It's not the protein – it's the fat that comes with the protein. If you don't believe this, try a little experiment. Tomorrow morning, have some pure protein powder with a glass of water for breakfast. You'll be hungry in an hour. The next day, have 4 oz (115 g) butter with a glass of water for breakfast. Call me when you feel hungry!

The best tip I can give you for successful low-fat cooking is to make foods wet! That's the golden rule of low-fat cooking. Eat your beans, peas and lentils as soups or top them with yoghurt sauces. Try cocktail sauces or lemon juice on salads and fish. Low-fat cottage cheese, yoghurt dressings, bananas, canned fish and lemon juice can be used to make sandwiches moist. Use mustard or ketchup instead of mayonnaise or butter on sandwiches. I'm sure one of my readers is saying, 'But ketchup has sugar in it!' Let me tell you, you'd have to spoon nearly 2 oz (50 g) of ketchup on your sandwich to equal the calories in 1½ teaspoons of mayonnaise. It's far better to use a little sugar to make foods tasty than to use a little fat. Even better than ketchup is a ripe, juicy tomato. Canned tomatoes have been the saviour of many a dry low-fat sandwich.

Fat also contributes to foods a flavour that is difficult to retain as we cut down on the fat. However, a little fat can carry a lot of flavour, and it isn't necessary to cut out fat entirely. Just find ways to reduce it. As mentioned earlier, the oil or butter in a recipe can easily be cut in half – or even to one-quarter of the suggested amount – without sacrificing flavour. Use skimmed or buttermilk when a recipe calls for whole milk. Substitute low-fat cottage cheese for the higher-fat cheeses. Yoghurt can replace soured cream. Mashed fruit, like bananas, or fruit juices can often replace much of the oil in baked goods.

You will find that you can still eat your favourite foods with just minor alterations. A 900-calorie dinner of chicken, mashed potatoes and gravy, asparagus with butter sauce, and salad with high-fat dressing can be reduced to 450 calories by skinning and grilling the chicken, adding a yoghurt sauce to the potatoes, lemon juice to the asparagus, and a low-calorie dressing to the salad.

Let's look at the ingredients for a lasagna recipe. Cooked according to this recipe, one serving would equal 670 calories because it is 51 percent fat. The following recipe looks almost unchanged. I kept the same ingredients so that the flavour would be almost identical. But because the fat is reduced to 32 percent a serving, it has only 495 calories. I also increased the fibre by substituting whole-wheat lasagna.

Lasagna

1 lb (450 g) Italian sausage
8 oz (225 g) minced beef
1 clove garlic
1 tablespoon basil
2 teaspoons salt
1 lb (450 g) tomatoes
6 oz (175 g) cans tomato
  purée
10 oz (300 g) lasagna
12 oz (350 g) full fat
  cottage cheese

6 oz (175 g) ricotta cheese
2 oz (50 g) grated Cheddar
  cheese
2 tablespoons chopped
  parsley
½ teaspoon pepper
2 eggs, beaten
116 (450 g) mozzarella
  cheese, thinly sliced

Lasagna (modified)

4 oz (115 g) Italian sausage
8 oz (225 g) lean minced beef
1 clove garlic
1 tablespoon basil
1 teaspoon salt
1 lb (450 g) tomatoes
6 oz (175 g) cans tomato
  purée
10 oz (300 g) whole-wheat
  lasagna
12 oz (350 g) low-fat cottage
  cheese

6 oz (175 g) part-skimmed
  ricotta cheese
2 oz (50 g) low-fat Cheddar
  cheese
2 tablespoons chopped
  parsley
½ teaspoon pepper
1 whole egg, 1 egg white,
  beaten
1 lb (450 g) part-skimmed
  mozzarella cheese, thinly
  sliced

Of course, you can change the recipe to a totally vegetarian dish, as in the third example, and further reduce calories to 345 a serving, at only 26 percent fat.

Modifying recipes by simply reducing the fat can have astonishing results. An average-sized chicken has 2000 calories. If you remove the skin, the calorie count goes down to 800! About 4 oz (115 g) chocolate pudding made with whole milk has 163 calories and is 28 percent fat. When it's made with skimmed milk, the calories drop to 130 and it becomes a 17 percent fat dessert. Ice cream is 50 percent fat, ice milk is 20 percent fat, and frozen yoghurt is 8 percent fat. Don't feel that you have to give up all your favourite foods. By cutting *down* the fat you can have your cake and eat it too! Well . . . almost.

Lasagna (vegetarian)

1 large onion, chopped

2 cloves garlic, minced

1 medium aubergine, diced

4 oz (115 g) mushrooms, sliced

2 tablespoons safflower oil

1 lb (450 g) canned tomatoes

1 8 oz (225 g) can tomato sauce

4 fl oz (120 ml) red wine

4 oz (115 g) grated carrot

1 oz (25 g) finely chopped parsley

2 teaspoons dried oregano

1 teaspoon dried basil

½ teaspoon salt

¼ teaspoon pepper

10 oz (300 g) wholemeal lasagna

1 lb (450 g) low-fat cottage cheese

8 oz (225 g) part-skimmed mozzarella cheese, thinly sliced

4 oz (115 g) grated Parmesan cheese

13

Fasting and Low-Calorie Dieting

Readers of *Fit or Fat?* will remember that I criticised fasting and low-calorie dieting because of the drastic muscle tissue loss that results from such programmes. Up to 30 percent of the weight lost will be muscle – the very tissue you need to burn up the food you eat. Furthermore, fasting and low-calorie dieting stimulate the activity of the lypogenic (fat-conserving) enzymes and depress lypolytic (fat-burning) activity. In simple terms, your metabolism slows down. You may be happy because you're losing weight, but with less fat-burning tissue (muscles) and increased fat-storing ability, you're going to gain fat more easily than ever before.

Lately the public has been bombarded by many new low-calorie diets. Proponents claim that these diets are good because they are consumed in special liquid or tablet mixtures and are produced in a laboratory whose personnel made sure all the essential vitamins and minerals were included. They claim that one need not worry about muscle protein loss because the diet's formula supplies the protein required by the body. So let's put some more nails in the low-calorie coffin!

1. It isn't weight loss that's important – it's fat loss that matters.

2. Many of the people we have tested who have lost weight on one of these diets have lost pounds of muscle

along with pounds of fat. This fact is countered with the argument that a loss of 1 lb (0.5 kg) of lean is worth it if you lose lots of fat. What concerns me is that the 1 lb (0.5 kg) of lean (protein) may include the enzymes that metabolize fats. It may include the antibody proteins that protect us from disease.

3. When muscle tissue loss occurs, glucose storage (as glycogen) in the muscles is reduced, augmenting any tendency toward diabetes.

4. The diets foster the idea that eating a set of chemicals put together in a laboratory is a healthy approach to life. While most of us are trying to eliminate chemicals – food additives, preservative, pesticides – from our food, these diets urge us to live on chemicals.

5. Despite loud claims from the salesmen, the diets are not new. They use the same tiresome idea (remember instant breakfast mixes and space food sticks?) that 300 to 400 calories per day are okay if taken in a magic formula.

6. They are *not* balanced diets! The brain demands blood glucose far in excess of that supplied by such a diet. The result is that the liver converts most of the protein in the diet, and possibly the vitamin C as well, to glucose. No diet is balanced when the liver wastes the nutrients in that diet by converting them to glucose.

7. The liver, which normally produces high-density lipoprotein (HDL) cholesterol (the good kind), shifts to the production of low-density lipoprotein (LDL) cholesterol (the kind implicated in arteriosclerosis) during a fast or radical low-calorie diet.

8. Those who lose weight on one of these diets can become 'counsellors', which appears to be a euphemism for sales-people. I find it particularly offensive that people with little or no nutrition background, unqualified to be counsellors, are answering newcomers' technical nutrition questions. This can be justified under the auspices of

'people helping people'. It can also be called the blind leading the blind.

9. Three to four hundred calories a day is drastic treatment, and there could be long-term effects as yet unknown. Remember the 'Last Chance Diet'? It was widely acclaimed until a few people died from it.

14

How to Lose Weight

Weight-loss programmes have been with us for years, yet even those designed by the best-trained professionals fail. People are getting fatter in spite of everything – so what does *weight*-loss mean? Is *weight* really what the fat person wants to lose? There is a joke in which one friend says to another, 'I know how you can lose ugly weight quickly; cut off your head.' It may be a dumb joke, but it makes a point. It's not weight that we need to lose, it's fat. If you think I'm splitting hairs, remember that weight-loss programmes don't work, and maybe if we get fussy and define exactly what we are trying to do we will find a better way to do it. While *weight loss* and *fat loss* may seem synonymous to you, it's the people who concentrate on fat loss who are successful. So let's talk sensibly from here on – not about losing weight but about losing fat.

Fat is lost from the body almost exclusively by being burned in muscle. You can't melt off fat in saunas, steam baths or plastic wraps. You can't rub off fat with vibrators, rolling machines or massages. You can't dissolve fat with a grapefruit diet, lecithin or any food supplement. Fat is released from storage sites into the blood to be carried to muscles. If the muscles don't burn the fat, it returns via the blood to be stored again in another fat depot. The only way you are ever going to get anywhere on a fat-loss programme is if your muscles burn the fat.

A healthy man's body is made up of about 40 percent

muscle; 32 percent muscle makes up a healthy woman's body. This 32 percent to 40 percent of the body performs 98 percent of the fat metabolism.

The big fault in most *weight*-loss schemes is that some of the lost weight is muscle, making the victim's body increasingly unable to burn fat. Don't make the mistake of thinking that a large weight loss is okay if *only* 1 lb of muscle is lost with it. That 1 lb (0.5 kg) is critical because any protein loss eventually decreases fat metabolism in muscle. What's the point of losing lots of weight if you are seriously impairing your body's ability to burn fat? Your bathroom scale is a pretty useless tool here because it cannot differentiate between amounts of fat and amounts of muscle. If you eat from the Target while exercising regularly, you will lose fat as you increase your ability to burn it.

> Exercise builds muscle;
> More muscle burns more fat;
> Less fat makes it easier to exercise;
> Exercise builds more muscle;
> More muscle burns more fat;
> And so on,
> And so on.
> 'The *Un*-Vicious Cycle of Fitness'
> Covert Truth No. 458-5

So never talk about *weight* loss again! Force yourself to use the term *fat* loss – and never adopt a programme that endangers body protein. Knowing that your muscles are the only place where excess fat can be burned, you mustn't start any diet programme that might impair your muscle efficiency. Stay on a good diet and exercise so your muscles will increase both their energy production and their heat production, enabling them to burn even more fat.

Now that you are concentrating on fat loss, you should find out how *much* fat you need to lose. You may *think* you know how much you need to lose, but you're thinking about weight again! You'll be much more successful if you find out how many actual pounds (kg) of fat your body has and how much of that you should lose. *You must have your body fat tested* to find out how many pounds (kg) of fat and how many pounds (kg) of lean you have. Your loss of muscle over the years will affect the amount of fat you should lose. Pretend you are a 10 stone (63.5 kg) woman who dreams of weighing 8 stone (50 kg). You feel you know exactly how much weight you want to lose. But what if your inactivity has caused muscle loss so that your muscles are soft even when you tighten them? Instead of being firm from exercise, your muscles have become flabby, lacking what is called muscle tone. Those soft muscles contain marbling fat that you should lose in addition to the obvious fat under your skin. You may need to lose 30 lbs (13 kg) of fat instead of 25 lb (11 kg).

The body-fat test tells you how much total fat you have, including the marbling in your muscles. It's a more responsible way of measuring how fat you are than by simply looking at your bulges or using the bathroom scales. You may be much fatter than you think because some of your fat *gain* has been masked by muscle *loss*. Unfortunately, people with poor muscle tone have trouble losing fat because poor muscle tone means poor fat burning. Your muscle can increase and decrease quite quickly. If you exercise during a fat-loss programme you may gain pounds (kg) of muscle as you lose pounds (kg) of fat! You'll think you are a failure at *weight* loss when, in fact, you are a success at *fat* loss.

Of all the people I have tried to help lose excess fat, the failures are those who won't have their fat tested. They think they know how fat they are and don't wish to be embarrassed by a test that would only confirm what they already know. Don't make this excuse! *Have your fat tested now!* The most accurate method is to be totally immersed in a tank of water. It's called hydrostatic immersion testing – available in America. It's inexpensive and it doesn't hurt. In fact, it's kind of fun. The only viable alternative to the water test is to be measured with skinfold calipers. The calipers aren't quite as accurate because they measure subcutaneous skinfold fat only. They are designed to *estimate* total body fat based on the measurement of subcutaneous fat.

Let me tell you how to use the information from a fat test. The results should be given to you as a percentage of body fat. Multiply your weight at the time of testing by that percentage to determine your *pounds* (kg) of body fat. Subtract your pounds (kg) of fat from your total body weight to determine your *pounds (kg) of lean*. Lean includes muscle, bone, skin, and all other fat-free tissue. For example, if you weigh 8½ stone (54 kg) and you are 30 percent fat, your results would look like this:

Total weight   = 8½ stone (54 kg)
Percentage of fat = 30%
lb (kg) of fat   = 36 lb (16 kg)
lb (kg) of lean   = 84 lb (38 kg)

To check your arithmetic, add your pounds (kg) of lean to your pounds (kg) of fat, making sure they equal your total weight.

For good health, a woman should not exceed 22 percent fat. Maximum allowable weight for a woman is figured by dividing her lean by 0.78, which is the same as saying that she shouldn't weigh more than her lean plus 22 percent. For our example, 84 lb (38 kg) of lean divided by 0.78 = 108 lb (49 kg). In other words, I feel that a woman with only 84 lb

(38 kg) of lean shouldn't weigh more than 7 st 10 lbs (49 kg) regardless of her height. Our 8½ stone (54 kg) woman needs to lose 12 lb (5.5 kg) of fat to be a healthy 22 percent.

A man shouldn't exceed 15 percent body fat for good health. Maximum allowable weight for a man is figured by dividing his lean by 0.85, so he shouldn't weigh more than his lean plus 15 percent.

Example

Weight	= 13 stone (82.5 kg)
Percentage of fat	= 20%
lb (kg) of fat	= 36 lb (16 kg)
lb (kg) of lean	= 144 lb (66.5 kg)
144 lb (66.5 kg) ÷ 0.85	
= Maximum allowable weight	= 12 stone (76 kg)
Needs to lose ⟶	11 lb (16 (5 kg)

Let's develop the numbers for our sample woman a little further. Suppose she is only five feet (1.52 m) tall and feels that 7 st 2 lb (45.5 kg) is what she really ought to weigh. We call this her fantasy weight.

Fantasy weight	= 7 st 2 lb (45.5 kg)
Actual weight	= 8½ stone (54 kg)
Percentage of fat	= 30%
lb (kg) of fat	= 36 lb (10 kg)
lb (kg) of lean	= 84 lb (38 kg)
Maximum allowable weight	= 7 st 10 lb (49 kg)

If you look at these figures carefully, you will uncover one of the main causes of failure in *weight*-loss programmes. People want to get from their actual weight to their fantasy weight regardless of whether the goal is realistic. To get to her fantasy weight of 7 st 2 lb (45.5 kg), our woman would have to lose 20 lb (9 kg) instead of the 12 lb (5.5 kg) of fat I recommend. In effect, she wants to be a 16-percent-fat woman which, in most cases, is unrealistic. She may protest that she would look better at 7 st 2 lb (45.5 kg). But 1 lb (0.5 kg) of fat takes up more space than 1 lb (0.5 kg) muscle. If you lose 1 lb (0.5 kg) fat while gaining 1 lb (0.5 kg) muscle, you will be smaller even though you weigh the same. If she got down to 7 st 10 lb (49 kg) through *fat* loss coupled with muscle firming, she would look better and wear a smaller dress size than if she went to 7 st 2 lb (45.5 kg) without muscle firming.

Don't focus on your fantasy weight! It is probably based on peer pressure or ridiculous height/weight charts. Have your body fat measured and calculate the number of pounds (kg) of fat you must lose to be a 22-percent-fat woman or a 15-percent-fat man. Then concentrate on losing fat while training your muscles to burn even more fat through exercise.

I hope you are now convinced of three important points:

1. Focus on fat loss rather than weight loss.
2. Muscle loss is to be avoided because it results in decreased fat burning.
3. Body-fat testing is the best way to design and monitor a fat-loss programme.

Now we come to the much-debated question of how many calories one should consume. There are 3500 calories in 1 lb (0.5 kg) of fat. If your muscles metabolized 500 more calories of fat per day than they usually do, in seven days you would theoretically burn off 3500 fat calories or 1 lb (0.5 kg). It seems logical to eat fewer calories per day so that the muscles will have to burn fat drawn from the fat cells. Unfortunately, it doesn't work quite that way for everyone. The explanation is a bit complicated, but let me give it a try.

Most people underestimate their calorie intake, so the following references to calories per day will seem high to many readers. There have been many studies in which volunteers were fed by dietitians who weighed and measured every morsel of food. The actual calorie totals ascertained by the dietitians were always much greater than the volunteers' estimates. Most women maintain their weight on 1200 to 2000 calories per day but feel that they eat less than that. For the sake of simplicity, I'm going to talk about women only, and only about those who are (or used to be) of average size. Excluding women who are exceptionally short or tall, large or small, we'll consider three groups:

Ms. Athlete: eats 2000 to 3000 calories per day; she maintains her weight.

Ms. Average: eats 1200 to 2000 calories per day: she may be near her correct weight or 30-40 lb (13.5-18 kg) overweight, but she maintains that weight.

Ms. Sedentary: eats fewer than 1200 calories per day; she may be happy with her weight or 100 lb (45.5 kg) overweight, but she maintains that weight.

Ms. Athlete really likes sports; she spends three to four hours a day, five days a week, exercising. She can eat 2500 calories without getting fat, while Ms. Sedentary gains weight on half that many calories. If Ms. Athlete eats 500 fewer calories a day, she can lose 1 lb (0.5 kg) of fat per week. Her athletic muscles are trained to burn stored fats, so her body will usually accept the 500-calorie decrease gracefully. She can lose fat easily, but Ms. Sedentary finds it difficult.

Ms. Sedentary claims to be 'very active' because she leads a busy life (gardening, chasing the kids) but, in fact, she isn't able to jog for twenty minutes, is nonathletic, and is not in tune with her body. At fewer than 1200 calories a day, she exists on the edge of basic metabolic needs. She will not tolerate a decrease of 500 calories a day well. Because her muscles don't burn fat well, she will lose much less than 1 lb (0.5 kg) *fat* per week. She may lose 1 lb (0.5 kg) of *weight*, but only part of it will be fat. The rest will be protein loss and the water loss that accompanies it. The fatter Ms. Sedentary is, the more apt she will be to lose muscle/water rather than fat.

When we consider Ms. Average, we flounder in a grey area because no one can tell her whether she is more like Ms. Sedentary or Ms. Athlete. Hence, no one can tell if a 500-calorie-per-day decrease will cause 1 lb (0.5 kg) fat loss or 1 lb (0.5 kg) muscle/water loss.

It has been assumed that a human body, used to consuming 2000 calories a day, when it is subjected to 1500 calories for a while will automatically draw 500 calories from fat stores. However, the body can say, 'I will live on fewer calories for a while', that is, decrease calorie requirement – and turn down metabolic rate. If your metabolic rate decreases during a 'weight'-loss programme, you will gain fat very quickly after the programme. Millions of people have lost 2-3 lb (1-1.5 kg) a week on radical low-calorie diets. Most of them are fatter today than they were before. Although 1 lb (0.5 kg) fat does contain 3500 calories, you do not always lose 1 lb (0.5 kg) of fat by eating 3500 fewer calories over a week or so.

My conclusion is that *no one* should strive for 1 lb (0.5 kg) *weight* loss per week. Ms. Athlete shouldn't because it's foolish to work so hard to obtain an athletic body and then expose it to such calorie stress. Ms. Athlete should be sufficiently in tune with her body to accept the gradual decrease in body fat that would come with a 200-calorie-per-day decrease.

My physician friends tell me that morbidly obese people – who have a lot of medical problems in addition to excess fat – *must* lose weight quickly 'for their health'. I disagree vehemently. Such people are invariably Ms. Sedentarys. In fact, the fatter you are, the less weight per week you should try to lose because your body tolerates sharp drops in calorie level less well. I urge those of you who are the most anxious to lose fat to make the least radical calorie reductions.

Athletic bodies seem to need and handle more calories than unfit bodies. Part of the reason is that fit people unconsciously move around more and produce more heat. But there is another reason. Fit people have more lean, the tissues that burn up fuel. Fit people, with firmer muscles, have a higher percentage of body lean because they have a lower percentage of body fat. Two people of the same age, sex, height and weight can have significantly different amounts of lean. Since it is the lean part of the body that burns up our food, it is tempting to tell people to find out how much lean they have (from a fat test) and then select a calorie level according to their amount of lean. Unfortunately, this method of selecting a calorie level isn't accurate either. Some people with large amounts of muscle metabolize calories slowly and some with small amounts of muscle metabolize quickly.

I have 140 lb (63.5 kg) of Lean Body Mass. One of my women co-workers has a small 90 lb (41 kg) Lean Body Mass. Our exercise habits are nearly identical. Theoretically, because I have two-thirds more more lean than she, I should be able to eat a lot more, but it doesn't work out that way. This woman often eats more than I do. We test her body fat frequently and know that it is stable at 20 percent in spite of her high calorie intake. Another female colleague has far more lean than the first woman, does double the daily exercise, yet gains fat if she doesn't maintain her calorie intake between 1500 and 2000 a day. Apparently, her higher muscle mass metabolizes food somewhat more slowly than the smaller woman's.

You can see from this example that even Lean Body Mass is not the key to determining caloric needs. The point I'm trying to make is that metabolism is very complicated and that no professional can assess your calorie needs more accurately than you yourself. Most people know their bodies well enough to know that they maintain weight on a certain number of calories and gain or lose if they exceed or decrease that amount. In spite of the fact that I consider 1000 to 1200 calories a day to be a minimal healthy level for women, many women gain weight on that many calories. These women are almost invariably Ms. Sedentarys, with a low percentage of body lean. They should concentrate less on reducing calories and more on increasing their lean. If you *gain* weight on fewer than 1000 calories (women) or 1400 calories (men), you need a tune-up. You have to increase calories to a minimum of 1200 (women) and 1700 (men) and do lots of aerobic exercise so your body will become a fat-burning machine.

If you want an estimate of your lean, try this. Tighten up your biceps and encircle it firmly with your free hand. Rotate your hand a bit so that you can feel the fat just under the skin outside the muscle. Then tighten your hand a bit more, testing the hardness of the muscle itself. For comparison, try this on several other people, including a couple of men and a teenage boy and girl. If you have been on low-calorie diets, you will probably find that your muscle seems soft no matter how hard you tighten it. This indicates a lot of fat or marbling in the muscle. It may sound odd but it means that there isn't much muscle in your muscle. Since muscle does about 98 percent of the body's fat burning, your fatty muscles account for your low calorie requirement.

We find that our most dedicated followers lose fat at about ½ percent fat per month. If you are 30 percent fat and want to be 20 percent, it will take twenty months, assuming that you eat 200 to 500 fewer calories a day than you have been consuming and do a minimum of one-half hour of aerobics every day. Frankly, those who lose ½ percent fat per month excercise for an hour every day. You may lose 1–3 lb (0.5–1.5 kg) of *weight* per week, but I implore you not to use weight as your criterion. Instead, have yourself fat tested periodically. Be sure to measure yourself from time to time. Both men and women show nice decreases in the waist measurement. Women, but not men, usually decrease nicely around the hips. A simple measuring tape can tell you more about fat loss than your bathroom scales.

Decrease your intake by a mere 200 calories and do some exercise. If you lose a little *weight* each week, that's a plus, but the significant changes will be internal and subtle, not measurable by anything so crude as a scale. You should *feel* different as the weeks go by. Most people experience a lightening of their step even if they have no weight loss. They know that something good is happening inside their bodies. Let's say you are 100 lb (45.5 kg) 'overweight' and your doctor urges you to lose 2–4 lb (1–2 kg) a week. *I* urge you not to follow his advice. He knows that your excess fat is bad for your health and he is sincerely trying to help you. But rapid weight loss raises more metabolic problems than it cures. Rapid weight loss also decreases metabolic rate so that one gets fatter than ever after the weight is lost.

In spite of all my cautions regarding excessive calorie reduction, the fact is that you still have to decrease calorie intake for effective fat loss. I feel that the following approach is the most practical one you will find. The easiest way to decrease calories and stay within the prescribed range is to decrease the fat in your diet. The easiest way to

93

do that is to count the number of fats you consume each day, by using the Target system. For the following chart to be really useful, you *must* have your body fat tested.

Recommended Daily Calories and Fats

	If Your Percentage Body Fat is OR		If You Don't Know Your Percentage of Body Fat* But You	You Should Eat			
				Calories/Day		Fats/Day	
	Men	Women		Men	Women	Men	Women
Cat. 1 (25% Fat Diet)	15% or less	22% or less	are satisfied with your present weight	2400– 2700	1700– 2000	No more than 15	No more than 11
Cat. 2 (20% Fat Diet)	16– 26%	23– 35%	want to lose 5–15 lb (2.5–6.5 kg)	1800– 2200	1400– 1700	8–10	6–8
Cat. 3 (10% Fat Diet)	27% or more	36% or more	want to lose more than 15 lb (6.5 kg)	1400– 1800	1000– 1400	3–4	2–3

* *Caution:* Using weight as your criterion is not smart. Read the text!

If you are not over 22 percent fat (women) or 15 percent (men), wish to maintain your present weight, and are a regular exerciser, the 25 percent fat diet of Category 1 is safe and healthy. The American Heart Association used to recommend a 30-percent-fat diet for everyone but dropped its recommendation to 20 percent when they realized that the majority of people do not fit into Category 1. The AHA seems to feel that all of us should eat as though we were as fat as the average person. I do not agree with their approach. Fit people's bodies can handle more dietary fat, and they deserve a category of their own. The Pritikin Diet makes the same error. It suggests that everyone should eat from Category 3, an extremely low-fat Spartan diet designed for obese heart patients.

A Category 1 woman could eat 2000 calories a day containing eleven fats. If she wanted to be less than 22 percent fat, however, she might put herself in Category 2 and eat 1700 calories and fewer fats. More typically, Category 2, at the 20 percent fat level, should be used by those who are moderately overfat and wish to lose 5–15 lb (2.5–6.5 kg). If you need to lose more than a stone (6.5 kg) of fat or have cardiovascular disease, you *must* stick to the 10 percent fat level of Category 3, which is, in effect, the Pritikin Diet.

The easiest way to eat a satisfying quantity of food without consuming too many calories is to count the fats in your diet. Analyse your daily food intake according to the Target, and you will soon find that it's easy to estimate calorie and fat intake by this method.

15

What is Fibre, Anyway?

Nobody knows! That's right, nobody knows exactly what fibre is. Scientists can't agree on a definition of fibre or even on how to measure the amount of it in food. If that isn't bad enough, we also aren't sure what it does. With all the confusion, why are nutritionists so sure we should eat it – and why should you believe them? Simply because a growing mountain of evidence shows that fibrous materials in food are beneficial. People who eat high-fibre diets have fewer intestinal tract problems like diverticulitis, spastic colon, haemorrhoids, constipation, and even colon cancer.

The basic idea of fibre is that there are substances in some foods which cannot be digested and therefore pass through the intestine out into the faeces. Obviously, if a substance passes right through like that, it won't supply calories. That doesn't mean the substance doesn't *contain* any calories, only that you aren't going to assimilate them. When horses eat hay, they get calories, but you and I could eat all the hay we wanted without gaining anything.

Suppose, then, that a person routinely eats 2 lb (1 kg) of food each day, mostly from the Meat and Milk groups. He would get very little fibre, digest and absorb most of what he eats, and produce limited faeces. If he were to get his 2 lb (1 kg) of food from the Bread and Cereal Group and the Fruit and Vegetable Group, he would produce greater faecal bulk with fewer calories absorbed, since many of the calories would be tied up in the fibre.

Fibre studies have increased dramatically over the last few years. A big push toward more dietary roughage occurred in the early 1970s, when scientists showed that members of African tribes who ate high-fibre diets had an extremely low incidence of colon cancer. Orientals also have a very low rate of colon cancer before they migrate to the United States. After eating the American high-fat/ low-fibre diet for one or two generations, Orientals contract cancer of the colon as frequently as Americans do. As a result of these findings, Americans started hunting for ways to bulk up their diets. It became popular to dump bran into all our high-fat recipes. Even cocktails were laced with bran. I have to admit that I was fooled into taking this simplistic approach myself. But then fibre in the diet was such a new concept that we didn't know that there are many kinds of fibre and that each one serves a different function. Today, adding bran to a food seems ridiculous to me, so I eat foods that have fibre in them to begin with.

When a lot of indigestible bulk is in the intestine, the transit time of the faecal contents is greatly speeded up. People on high-fibre diets digest and eliminate a meal in fourteen hours, as compared with the forty-eight-hour interval it takes to move the usual high-fat meal through the colon. Does the transit time of food through the colon really matter? You bet it does! In order to digest fat, the liver produces bile, which goes into the intestine where it breaks down fat molecules. Bile is an acid that can irritate and abrade the intestinal lining if allowed to remain in constant contact with it. Most scientists believe that this constant irritation from bile acids give rise to intestinal abrasions and sores, which can eventually lead to cancer. Thus, if food moves quickly through the colon, the bile acids will also be moved through quickly. Additionally, a high-fibre diet usually means a lower-fat diet. If not much fat is present in the first place, then not much bile is produced.

Colon cancer, the number two cancer killer in America, prompts many medical people to worry about those who suffer repeated bouts of diarrhoea, constipation, or other seemingly mild colon conditions. It's possible that some or all of these conditions may lead to cancer and, luckily, most can be alleviated by fibre in the diet. Greater faecal bulk and faster transit time greatly reduce constipation and the haemorrhoids that result from it. And, though the reasoning is less obvious, the same high-fibre diet can stabilize a spastic colon and diarrhoea. 'Faster transit time!' the diarrhoea victim exclaims. 'That's the *last* thing I need!' In diarrhoea, too much unabsorbed free water in the intestine causes muscular spasm and violent emptying of faecal contents. The gelatinous structure of fibre can absorb the excess water and fill out the intestinal cavity with a more solid mass. If you've had an irritable colon for years, the sudden introduction of a high-fibre diet may worsen the condition. Your colon may be so used to high fat and low fibre that it doesn't know how to handle the added bulk. Introduce fibre very slowly, over a long period of time.

The ability of fibrous foods to fill out the intestinal cavity has also proved beneficial to people suffering from diverticulitis. In this condition, the lining of the large intestine has small outcroppings in which food and bacteria get entrapped, leading to inflammation and infection. The gelatine and bulk produced by a fibre diet tend to smooth and clean out these small pockets.

Cellulose and hemicellulose, the fibres responsible for bulk and fast transit time, are found mainly in the grains and cereals and in vegetables. When high-roughage diets first became popular, the cellulose and hemicellulose fibres were stressed, and that's why it seemed so practical to sprinkle bran (the fibre found in wheat) on everything. Today, scientists have discovered exciting qualities about the fibres found in fruits and in beans, peas and lentils.

These fibres – such as pectin and guar – have a profound effect on blood glucose and the insulin response. In fruits and beans and peas, pectin and other fibres tie up sugar molecules so that they are absorbed very slowly into the bloodstream. Cellulose-type fibres do not seem to do this as well. The result is that blood sugar rises more slowly when pectin is included in a meal. This, in turn, elicits a low insulin response, which is good news for those with diabetes, the third most common disease in the United States. In the past, doctors treated diabetics by removing most carbohydrates from their diets. The theory was that if there were no glucose molecules in the food, the pancreas wouldn't have to produce insulin. This is another example of treating the symptom rather than the cause. Today, most doctors advise diabetic patients to avoid the simple carbohydrates but encourage them to eat complex carbohydrates. Unless the patient is insulin-dependent, the pancreas can usually handle the trickle of glucose introduced by fibrous foods.

As an aside, it's interesting to note that in the late 1960s diabetic patients were often told not to exercise. Today the opposite is true. Gentle aerobic exercise is encouraged because it makes the muscle tissue more receptive to insulin. (Unfit muscles tend to reject insulin.)

The physical form of fibrous food also influences glucose and insulin response. Raw fruits, vegetables, and beans and peas elicit the mildest response. Cooking, grinding, puréeing, and juicing produces sharper rises in blood glucose and in insulin. In fact, the purée or juice of a fruit or vegetable produces glucose and insulin responses almost identical to those of eating an equal load of pure glucose. The fibre is there all right, but it has been so 'refined' that it no longer does its job. I recommend eating a whole fruit or vegetable rather than drinking the juice. The fibre from one orange gives fewer calories, greater satiety, less sugar, and more beneficial effects than one glass of orange juice made from four oranges.

Foods such as dried beans and lentils have a unique characteristic not seen in other plant products. If they are cooked but eaten whole, the glucose and insulin responses are very mild. If cooked and minced or puréed, the glucose response is much higher, but the insulin response is virtually identical to the one elicited by the whole bean. In other words, beans evoke particularly mild insulin responses regardless of their physical form. Scientists speculate that the high protein content of dried peas, beans and lentils may be the cause. In any case, this makes beans, peas and lentils an ideal food for diabetics, whose metabolism cannot afford to undergo sudden and sharp rises in insulin production.

I have discussed only a few of the known benefits of fibre in the diet; more are being postulated all the time. Nonetheless, scientists continue to argue about fibre. What is it chemically? How does it work? Is it really the agent responsible for observed metabolic effects? In spite of these unknowns, we *do* know that obesity is our number one health problem, and a high-fibre diet is the second best way to attack it.

16

How Much Fibre Should We Eat?

There are so many different kinds of fibre – pectin, cellulose, hemicellulose, etc. – that it is difficult to give a definitive answer. It is not only impossible to state how much of each fibre we need, but we also don't know how much of each fibre is present in foods. Years ago, when fibre wasn't considered to be all that important, 'crude fibre' analysis was done by people in laboratories scattered all over the world. Their techniques were different and their results subject to prejudice, yet all the numbers were gathered together in one collection of nutrition tables that we still use today. Their basic technique was to prepare a food as if it were going to be eaten, then to 'digest' it with various acid and alkaline solutions that were supposed to mimic human digestion. The part of the food that wasn't digested was called crude fibre. The drawback to these early studies was that laboratory chemicals couldn't imitate human enzyme processes, and most foods were overdigested. The new studies, which are more similar to human digestion, give us what is called dietary fibre. Apparently, the chemicals used for the early crude-fibre analysis were too strong, leaving much less undigested fibre residue than our intestines do. In other words, there is a lot more fibre in foods than the early tables indicate. Most people would agree from personal observation that corn on the cob leaves a far greater undigested residue than the 1 percent listed in the tables.

Current studies on fibre content are now done on volunteers. The tests are more accurate, but more time-consuming, and, as you can imagine, not exactly pleasant for those who undergo them. As a result, comparatively few foods have been reanalysed. Of those that have been, most show two to nine times as much fibre as the earlier studies. When you read about fibre, be sure to distinguish between the low crude-fibre results of yesteryear and the much larger dietary fibre figures of today.

Variations in dietary fibre measurements reflect the physical form of the food. For example, the less the refinement of the grain in breads and cereals, the greater their dietary fibre. Vegetables and fruits have a lot of water, which effectively dilutes the dietary fibre, thus giving smaller values. As mentioned earlier, the dried beans, peas and lentils are unusual because they yield high dietary fibre regardless of the degree of refinement.

The average person on a typical high-fat/low-fibre diet consumes about 10 to 12 grams of dietary fibre a day. The African studies showed average intakes of 100 grams a day! Clearly, if we expect our bodies to initiate the intestinal and blood chemistry changes discussed earlier, we must consume many more fibrous foods.

After this discussion, you will realize that the fibre quantities shown in the Appendix are far from precise. They represent my best interpretation of the old and the new data available. Dietary fibre is usually reported in grams. However, the word *gram* implies an accuracy that is not warranted, so I refer to 'fibres' in a food. In the Target system, one fibre approximates 1 gram of dietary fibre. But because of conflicting data, this is a rough calculation. I have tried to err on the low side so that if you eat fifteen fibres, in most cases you'll be getting more than 15 grams of fibre.

I advise people to aim for a minimum of fifteen fibres a

day. If you eat the recommended four servings from the Fruit and Vegetable Group and the four from the Bread and Cereal Group, you'll be guaranteed at least sixteen fibres a day, just about the necessary minimum. Then, by adding a dried bean, pea or lentil dish three to four times a week, you'll assure yourself of getting all the fibre you need.

17

Do We Need to Take Vitamins?

Every time I lecture, someone asks me, 'Do I need to take vitamins?'

The question is ridiculous – obviously we have to take vitamins. Vitamins, by definition, are chemicals, taken orally in miscroscopic amounts, that are required to sustain life or *vita*. The real question is whether we need to take vitamins in addition to those in our food. You may object to my answer, claiming that it should have been obvious in the original question. If one phrases the question responsibly, however, it is easy to frame a responsible answer. *It depends on what one eats!* If one eats very little food, one is not likely to get enough vitamins. Similarly, if one selects foods of low nutrient density, one is not likely to get enough vitamins. Nine-month-old babies who receive only bottled milk tend to get plenty of calories but no iron at all. Hence, they get fat but anaemic. An adult woman who lives on cottage cheese, yoghurt, salads, vegetables, and fruits might easily do the same – get fat and anaemic. If this woman took supplementary iron pills, she might be fat but not anaemic.

It is estimated that of all the calories an ordinary person eats, 45 percent come from fat, 15 percent from sugar, and another 15 percent from white flour. In other words, approximately 70 percent of our calories come from foods containing precious few vitamins and minerals. That means we expect to derive nutrition from 30 percent of our food. Therefore, a typical diet at the 2000-calorie level gives 1400 empty calories and only 600 calories of significant nutritional value. This implies that 30 percent of our calorie intake supplies 100 percent of our nutrition.

If you are a social drinker, you must add approximately another 10 percent of empty calories to your total, expecting to get vitamins and minerals from only 20 percent of your food.

If you are on a 1000-calorie (or less) weight-loss diet, it is impossible to get the necessary nutrition no matter how nutritious the diet may appear to be or how many vitamins and minerals are added to it. Calories are just as essential to life as vitamins or protein. When calories fall below about 1700 a day for men, or 1200 a day for women, the liver sees to it that some of the vitamins get consumed as fuel rather than used as vitamins, thereby producing a vitamin deficiency. Even a carefully manufactured diet, supplemented with the most nutritious-sounding ingredients, will be vitamin deficient if calories are too low.

It's popular to criticize our food supply, suggesting that it is impossible to get enough vitamins from our foods. Critics claim that because vegetables are grown on depleted soils and shipped long distances, they are less nutritious than the fresh vegetables of our ancestors. The fact is, of course, that our ancestors didn't get *any* fruits or vegetables when they were out of season. Neither did they get quick-fresh-frozen orange juice, which retains all its vitamin C until it's made back into juice, at which time it starts losing Vitamin C at the same rate as fresh orange juice.

It seems to me it's better to eat the great variety of available fruits and vegetables all the time, as we can today, than the fresh fruits and vegetables that were available to our ancestors two months a year. I'm just old enough to remember the wizened-up, dead-looking fruits and vegetables that my parents tried to preserve in our fruit cellar. I can also remember how bare the vegetable section of our market looked in winter. The claim that we got more nutritious fruits and vegetables in the 'old days' makes me laugh. Let's stop 'blame shifting'! There are plenty of good foods to eat. If you select a high-fat, high-sugar, white-flour, alcohol diet, your vitamin deficiency can only be blamed on you. Most researchers agree that all of us *could* get plenty of vitamins and minerals if we *would* eat properly.

To answer the initial question, 'Do I need to take vitamins?' the answer is yes. Eat enough food of high quality and you will get plenty of vitamins. But do we need to ingest vitamin/mineral supplements in addition to our food? If you consume a typical Western diet, the answer is yes! You will not get sufficient vitamins and minerals, and you should take vitamin/mineral supplements.

So if your diet is low in vitamins and minerals because it is unbalanced or low in calories or consists of empty-calorie selections, you will want to consider supplements.

I like to think about vitamin dosage on five levels:

1. Vitamin toxicity
2. Subclinical toxicity
3. So-called subclinical deficiency
4. Recommended Daily Allowance (RDA)
5. Deficiency disease

We know the most about vitamin dosage at Level 5 because rampant vitamin deficiency in the early 1900s spiked the original vitamin research and the first vitamin was discovered. The word *vitamin* wasn't even a word before then because we didn't know that there were essential food chemicals in microscopic amounts. Before that, it was thought that one needed only to eat 'enough' food – eat for bulk – satisfy hunger and all would be well.

Once the concept of essential food chemicals was established, an academic rush was on to discover in foods other chemicals that are essential to life. Scientists were quick to put animals on deficient diets, and scientific papers regarding deficiency syndromes of one vitamin or mineral after another proliferated. It was relatively easy to establish the dietary level of a vitamin/mineral that would produce a deficiency disease. Vitamin C, however, fooled the researchers for a long time, because most of their laboratory animals didn't get scurvy. Most lab animals make their own vitamin C, so they don't need it in their diets and for them *it isn't a vitamin.*

A note in passing – pangamic acid, widely sold as vitamin B_{15}, does not occur naturally in foods, is not essential to life, and is not a vitamin for human beings. It hasn't been shown to be useful to any animal.

Research quickly established the dosage necessary to prevent deficiency disease. By applying some sophisticated maths, one can establish the dosage necessary to prevent human deficiency disease, and it was tempting at first to accept these levels as adequate. The minimum daily requirement, or MDR, was established, but put aside as less than adequate under such circumstances as stress, disease or pregnancy.

Then the RDAs evolved. I put them at Level 4. The vitamin merchants claim that the Recommended Daily Allowances are set by the government. This is not true! They are, in fact, a consensus of professors of nutrition the world over. In many cases the RDA is more than double the amount necessary to prevent deficiency disease. In other words, the RDA of a vitamin or mineral is enough to prevent deficiency disease even in individuals with conditions that greatly increase their need over the average person's.

Naturally, researchers also tried giving laboratory

animals very *high* doses of these exciting substances. After all, if a little increases one's *vita,* then a lot might produce superhumans or perhaps make us live longer. From these studies, we get dosage levels that I put at Level 1 on my chart. Level 1, 'toxicity', should be self-explanatory, but the concept is played down by the vitamin pushers. When I was a teenager, cod liver oil was so popular that parents were forcing it on their kids and the resultant vitamin A and vitamin D toxicity deaths became a national scandal. All the fat-soluble vitamins (A, D, E, K) are stored in the body's fat deposits so that toxic levels are easily attained. Entire books have been written about the symptoms of toxicity from fat-soluble vitamins.

The B vitamins and vitamin C, because they are water-soluble, are quickly excreted in the urine, making overdosage less likely.

Vitamin A toxicity is particularly interesting: 100,000 International Units (IU) per day produce brain damage and death in laboratory rats. (For simplicity, I use the human equivalent of the rat dosage.) Naturally, researchers wanted to know what dosage the rats could take without getting such drastic effects. They kept diminishing the dose until, at 50,000 IU per day, the rats suffered no ill effects at all. With 5000 IU being the RDA level and 100,000 IU the severely toxic, 50,000 IU seemed to be a maximum safe dosage. One university professor, however, wanted to be absolutely sure, so he bred rats that received 50,000 IU per day to see whether their offspring would show ill effects. The offspring were fine! So, feeding them the same diet, he let them grow up, breed, and produce their own offspring. The third generation showed teratological (monster) effects – predominantly brain damage and hydrocephalus. It is apparent that while loading up on vitamins may seem to be beneficial, such 'self-medication' could, in fact, produce changes in the body that could have harmful results years or generations later.

In any case, 50,000 IU of vitamin A, just tenfold the RDA, is easily attained by taking the vitamin A pills available in many stores.

Humans have a natural tendency to want more of something that seems to be good for them. (If one is good, two is better.) So it's a natural temptation to try vitamin/ mineral pills 'just in case'. Because they occur naturally in our food, we think they can't hurt us. But we can see from the discussion on toxicity that they *can*.

The big problem comes when we move into the grey area between the blatantly toxic Level 1 of a vitamin and the clinically useful RDA Level 4. People who take lots of vitamin/mineral supplements claim that they are necessary to guard against subclinical disease (Level 3). But it's possible that they may be producing subclinical toxicity (Level 2).

Even drugs that are considered effective and safe carry warnings. Although vitamins occur naturally in our food, when you take them as supplements you are treating them as drugs, and they *do* have definite side effects. Raising the dosage may increase the benefits, but it may also increase the side effects. As with most drugs, it's impossible to be sure that for every person who takes the drug the benefits are worth the side effects.

Ten milligrams of vitamin C per day produces Level 5 scurvy. Thirty milligrams of vitamin C per day prevents scurvy in otherwise healthy people. Sixty milligrams of vitamin C per day (the RDA) prevents scurvy in almost everyone – even those with weird extenuating circumstances. Linus Pauling pushes 600 to 1000 milligrams of vitamin C per day to ward off colds. Many dentists recommend similarly high levels of the vitamin because they feel that patients' gums become healthier and heal better. Nutritionists criticize Pauling for his unscientific method, explaining that such large doses of vitamin C can't do any good because they simply pass through the body, appearing in the urine in one hour. Pauling counters with the theory that the extra vitamin C does good things on the way through. Who is right? I don't know yet. But I do know that 600 milligrams per day is ten times the RDA and may produce side effects more serious than the mild side effects already recognized. Pauling recommends 10 grams or 10,000 milligrams of vitamin C per day if you feel a cold coming on. This high level is approximately one hundred times the RDA and, although I can't prove anything, I feel intuitively that it is ridiculous. It takes only ten times the RDA of vitamin A to produce third-generation brain damage, yet Pauling urges one hundred times the RDA for vitamin C. Even though vitamin C is water-soluble, it seems to me that doses at one hundred times the RDA are well into Level 2 or 3. Yes, it might knock out a cold; so might five swallows of chloroform or three of carbon tetrachloride.

If you do increase vitamin C intake when you notice the first symptoms of a cold, you should be aware of the 'rebound effect'. The liver produces an enzyme that breaks down excess vitamin C, and increased vitamin C intake increases the production of this enzyme. Many people stop taking the extra vitamin C when a cold is gone. The enzyme in the liver, which increased to high levels during the megadoses of vitamin C, then finds it has nothing to do and thus breaks down all the vitamin C you take. It will even break down the vitamin C that you *do* need. This throws you into a vitamin C deficiency and perhaps sets you up for a relapse of the cold. (By the way, megadoses of vitamin C produce an antihistamine effect on the body. People who claim that vitamin C cleared up their runny noses could have obtained the same results by using over-the-counter remedies. The vitamin C did not 'cure' the cold – it alleviated the symptoms.)

The rebound effect of vitamin C makes me wonder

whether large dosages of other vitamins might cause negative effects as well. It seems odd to me that those who are quickest to denounce a particular food preservative, even if it has never been shown to produce side effects, are the quickest to take vitamins or minerals at Level 2 and 3 dosages. The advantages are vague and speculative at best. The toxic side effects are more probable. It makes good sense to me to consume dosages of vitamins that occur normally in foods. Would you eat twenty-four oranges a day? That's the number you would need to get the 2 grams of vitamin C pushed by many health food advocates. A second reason for getting your vitamins from food is that it's impossible to overdose on those. You couldn't eat enough carrots to get vitamin A toxicity. Even if you could, the vitamins found naturally in food do not produce the same toxic effects that vitamins in pills do. Finally, there may be vitamins and minerals as yet undiscovered. You are far more likely to get them from foods than from manufactured pills.

In the final analysis, I feel that any discussion of the proper amount or kind of vitamin/mineral supplement misses the point. If you eat right, you can get more than enough of both – and decrease the empty-calorie fats, sugars, white flour, and alcohol that are making us fat.

18

What About Salt?

The controversy over sodium invariably arises during each of my lectures. My usual answer sounds flippant: 'Let's worry about the fat now, and we'll get the salt out of the diet next year'. I suppose this makes some people mad, but let's think seriously about it for a moment.

Recent evidence shows that criticism about the amount of salt – or rather, the sodium – in the diet may be overemphasized. Sodium is certainly implicated in high blood pressure (hypertension), but body fat may have more to do with how a person handles sodium than previously thought. It goes back to my old premise. If you're fat, your body will react to certain environmental infringements differently than if you're fit. As a rule, a fat body handles sodium poorly; a fit body handles it well. So if you are fat and out of condition, you should certainly be careful about your sodium intake, just as you should be careful about your vitamin/mineral intake, your sugar consumption, your fat consumption, and so on, and so on. A fit body is a finely tuned mechanism that can handle an occasional overload of fat, sugar, salt, or whatever.

You could be saying, 'This may be true, but even a fit body shouldn't be subjected to constant nutritional abuse'. And you're right! So here are some basic guidelines for sodium intake.

I recommend that people in normal health consume no more than 2000 milligrams of sodium a day. Two thousand milligrams is the equivalent of 1 teaspoon of salt. Most food labels today list the sodium content of the product. Select brands that are lowest in sodium. Focus on the word *sodium* on the label. The ingredient's rank on the label will give you an idea of its relative amount in the food. (First ingredient is the most abundant, second is the second most abundant, and so on.) The word *sodium* should stand out like a red flag, but don't be fooled by such words as *disodium phosphate* or *monosodium glutamate*. They are just as bad.

Take the salt cellar off the dinner table.

Watch out for sodium in medications. Some antacids contain more than one-quarter of the daily recommended amount of sodium in each dosage.

Water softeners often contain a lot of sodium. If you are concerned about your sodium intake, avoid using softened water for cooking and drinking. But if you substitute bottled water, be sure to check it for sodium content – some bottled waters have a lot of it.

Avoid or limit your eating of such obviously salty foods as potato crisps, pretzels, crackers, salted fish, salted nuts, popcorn, pickles, olives, sauerkraut, luncheon meats and processed soups.

If you eat in or near the bull's-eye of the Target Diet you don't have to be concerned about sodium because you won't find much there. Unless you destroy the diet with salt at the dinner table, Target Diet foods are extremely low in sodium. Where is the salt in the Meat Group – in the beans, or in the bacon? Where is the salt in the Bread and Cereal Group – in the wholemeal bread, or in the preservatives and additives in the savoury crackers and party snacks?

It turns out that my remark about attacking the salt problem next year is not an irresponsible answer after all. Learn how to eat correctly *now*. Get fit *now*. Then salt *won't* be a problem next year.

19

Protein Quantity and Quality

The RDA (Recommended Daily Allowance) for protein is only 44 grams per day for women and 56 grams per day for men. Most people on the typical high-meat-and-milk-product diet exceed these levels by severalfold. The male students in my college classes rarely consume less than three times the RDA for protein. We have a fascination for protein that approaches the ridiculous. Even hair sprays and shampoos are sold on the basis of their protein content. Nutrition studies are misleading, because we must study nutrients by giving animals too *little* and noting side effects. Then, when we get around to it, we give animals too *much* and note the side effects. The public has so often heard that it's bad to have too little protein that it can't believe we could have too much.

Unfortunately, a growing body of evidence indicates that consuming too much protein is not only foolish; it can be harmful. As dietary protein is increased in excess of the RDA, calcium excretion in the urine is increased. Three hundred to 400 milligrams of calcium per day is considered to be plenty in most countries, but in the United States, where dietary protein is so high, scientists believe we need 800 milligrams per day to compensate for the calcium loss caused by excess protein. In Third World countries, average daily intake of calcium is less than half the U.S. RDA for calcium, yet mothers nurse their young for twenty months or more without any apparent ill effect. Furthermore, women in these Third World countries have much less bone loss (osteoporosis), despite what we would call a low-calcium diet. Doctors in America often prescribe even more than the RDA of calcium for postmenopausal women to prevent osteoporosis. Why should U.S. women have calcium loss on 1000 milligrams calcium per day and black African women have almost none despite only 300 milligrams per day and lengthy breast feeding? The answer seems to be that a high-protein diet with its attendant very high calcium/phosphorus ratios fosters calcium loss. High-protein diets and high-protein drinks can be bad for you!! Excess protein can be considered toxic – there are bad side effects.

Note also that Third World dietary protein comes primarily from vegetable sources, not meat or milk products. This makes the issue even more interesting, since so many people feel that vegetable and grain proteins are inadequate because they are incomplete. We all know that vegetable proteins lack some of the essential amino acids, making these proteins less usable. Studies have shown that 24 grams per day of meat protein is plenty for most people, whereas 25 grams per day is required if wheat protein is substituted for meat and 31 grams per day if soy protein is used. Note, however, that all of these levels are only one-half the RDA. In other words, the RDA is double what we really need, regardless of the source. Furthermore, the studies always use only one protein at a time, while few people actually eat that way. When account is taken of the fact that people usually vary their dietary protein and eat more than one protein at each meal, the protein requirement diminishes and source becomes almost unimportant.

The original studies, which indicate that mixing proteins to enhance quality must occur at each meal, made use of purified amino acids rather than actual proteins. More recent studies show that a mixture of purified amino acids that is supposed to simulate a particular protein is not utilized as well as the actual protein itself. Incomplete proteins are not as poorly utilized as once thought, for two reasons. When an incomplete protein is eaten, some of the missing essential amino acids are supplied by sloughed off intestinal lining cells and other endogenous breakdown products. Additionally, food protein stays in the gut much longer than purified amino acids, so that proteins consumed at one meal are often available to mix and match with proteins in a later meal. It was previously thought that the eight essential amino acids had to be consumed within an hour and a half of each other or they wouldn't be utilized. The book *Diet for a Small Planet* urged us all to mix our plant proteins *very carefully* at every meal or we would be protein-deficient; this is clearly not an important issue in light of more recent studies. But please don't think I'm too critical of *Diet for a Small Planet*. The book's discussion of world food problems, and of diet adjustments that you and I should make to alleviate these problems, is excellent.

In underdeveloped countries, protein supply is marginal, not because protein quality is low but because dietary protein of whatever source is accompanied by limited calories. In these countries, starvation is primarily a carbohydrate problem leading to the misuse of limited protein because proteins are converted to carbohydrate when calories are low. Even if the normal protein requirement *is* met, proteins are converted to carbohydrate if calorie requirement is *not* met. This also occurs in affluent countries when people try to lose weight on diets that claim to have adequate protein in spite of their low calories, such as the Cambridge Diet, the Atkins Diet, and the Stillman Diet. In biochemistry there is an age-old phrase, 'carbohydrate spares protein'. It seems odd to me

119

that half of our population is afraid it isn't getting enough protein, while the other half searches for severe starvation diets of 300 to 900 calories, which endanger the little protein they eat. Whatever happened to the well-balanced diet and common sense?

The conclusion has to be that protein malnutrition in the West is almost impossible because:

1. We get plenty of calories (if we choose to).
2. Plant proteins are better than we thought.
3. Most people eat two or more proteins at each meal.
4. Most people vary their proteins from day to day.
5. All essential amino acids do *not* have to be included at each meal.

We eat much more protein than we need! Such high protein ingestion causes bone calcium loss as well as liver and kidney stress from the excess nitrogen, ammonia, and urea that must be excreted. If you are consuming a correct number of calories each day (at least 1700 for men and 1200 for women) but are getting excess protein, try eating more calories from complex carbohydrates and fewer from protein.

Take a look at the two lunches below. Notice that the greasy fast-food lunch supplies all the protein a woman needs for the entire day, but at the expense of 755 calories, 51 percent of which come from fat. In contrast, the low-fat/high-fibre lunch supplies almost an equal amount of protein with many fewer calories, only 15 percent of which come from fat.

Fast-Food Lunch
1 cheeseburger
chips
1 glass whole milk

Low-Fat/High-Fibre Lunch
1 tuna fish (brine-packed) sandwich
Low-calorie mayonnaise
1 apple
1 carrot
1 glass skimmed milk

Food	Grams Protein	Food	Grams Protein
3 oz (75 g) hamburger	23	3 oz (75 g) tuna fish	24
1 oz (25 g) cheese	7	Low-calorie mayonnaise	—
1 bun	4	2 slices wholemeal bread	6
chips	2	1 apple	1
8 fl oz (250 ml) whole milk	8	1 carrot	1
		8 fl oz (250 ml) skimmed milk	8

Total grams of protein	= 44	Total grams of protein	= 40
Total calories	= 755	Total calories	= 450
Percentage of calories from fat	= 51	Percentage of calories from fat	15

20

Cholesterol, Heart Attack and Arterial Disease

A heart attack is usually the result of another problem. The other problem is arteriosclerosis – a disease of the arteries. Before a heart attack occurs, there is often nothing wrong with the heart. But the arteries can become so sick that they literally 'attack' the heart by shutting off the needed blood and oxygen. The heart, after all, is a muscle; like any other muscle it has a blood supply. Unlike other muscles, the heart muscle can't rest if its blood supply is interrupted. Three main arteries deliver blood to the heart; typically, only one of these arteries suffers sudden blockage. Therefore, only one segment of the muscle is attacked. This could be compared to a severe bruise in any other muscle. *If* the heart could rest, heart attacks wouldn't be so bad!

Imagine running in the dark and hitting your leg on the corner of a table. You might be able to continue running – but only on one leg. Or imagine striking an equally hard blow to the thigh muscles of several people. The large-muscled individual might be able to run with minor pain. The small individual, having a proportionately larger amount of muscle damaged, might not even be able to walk. Similarly, if there is sudden blockage in a tiny artery feeding a small segment of the heart, the person might feel little or no pain, recover in a few moments, and the heart attack would go undiagnosed. Suppose, however, that the other arteries to the heart are narrowed by plaque (fat deposits) and an attack occurs while the victim is in the middle of an exercise. The heart would be so compromised that the 'small heart attack' would become the final straw, the pain too much, and the heart would stop.

Arteriosclerosis compromises the heart by gradually narrowing blood vessels and then *attacks* the heart by throwing off a chunk of fatty material that floats a little way and then suddenly plugs an artery completely. A stroke is pretty much the same thing. One of the arteries that lead to the brain shuts off, and part of the brain dies from lack of oxygen.

A trip to an autopsy room might help you to visualize arteriosclerotic plaque. A doctor could demonstrate on any artery, but for our purposes we'll have him remove the largest one, the aorta, which is about the same size and thickness as an ordinary garden hose. We'll have our imaginary doctor cut out about a foot of the hoselike aorta, lay it on a table, and then slit it lengthwise so you can look at the inside. The layman, having heard all about fatty cholesterol plaques in arteries, would expect to see chunks of yellowish material on the inside of the aorta. Not so. The wall appears to be very slippery and smooth. This would be true in any artery, large or small. Suppose the doctor has you run your thumb up the inside of the aorta. I know this sounds gruesome, but picture it in your mind. Your thumb will go along pretty smoothly for about 1 inch (2.5 cm) or so, and then it will get stuck, as if there were a chunk of something under the surface. As you push your thumb over this chunk it will make a clicking or crackling noise. As you continue to run your thumb up the inside of the artery you will come across several of these chunks or bumps that crackle. If the doctor were to cut the aorta crosswise he could show you that these lumps are fatty cholesterol plaques. Under a microscope you would find that these plaques are composed mainly of saturated fat, which is the

124

same kind of fat that rings a good steak. A small percentage of the plaque is composed of crystals of cholesterol, which break easily and are responsible for the clicking noise you heard.

The fact that the plaques in the arteries are composed of saturated fat and cholesterol has been especially profitable for the makers of various unsaturated vegetable oils. Although there is evidence that the cholesterol in your blood seems to go down when you consume poly-unsaturated fats (like vegetable oils) it would be foolish to conclude that unlimited consumption is safe. For one thing, scientists now suspect a link between poly-unsaturated fats and cancer. For another thing, your body is composed of saturated fat – as an animal you naturally are not going to have polyunsaturated or vegetable fats in your tissues. So if you eat a polyunsaturated fat, what do you think is going to happen to it? Of course! It will be converted into a saturated fat. Overall, the consumption of polyunsaturated fats seems to be safer than saturated fats. But emphasis should be placed on reducing total fat intake and then, if you simply have to have some fat, stick to the polyunsaturated ones.

Blood cholesterol typically ranges between 120 and 300 milligrams percent (milligrams in 100 millilitres). Most doctors feel you are at a safe level if it is under 220 milligrams percent. I feel better when people are under 180 milligrams percent. I should caution you, however, that many factors induce temporary changes in cholesterol level, and there can be marked fluctuations in a healthy person. For this reason, at least three readings should be taken over a three- to four-month period for a determination of one's average cholesterol level.

You may be able to find out from your doctor what percentage of your cholesterol is high-density lipoprotein (HDL) and what percentage low-density lipoprotein

(LDL). Cholesterol is a fat and as such can't dissolve in the blood any better than oil dissolves in water. Cholesterol has to 'fool' the blood into accepting it, which it does by coating itself with some protein (called lipoprotein, where *lipo* stands for fat). You have to picture all of this on a microscopic level, but when a relatively large chunk of fat and cholesterol get together and get wrapped up in a protein, it is very much like a fat person. When a fat person is in water he floats quite easily, and we say he is not very dense – he has low density. These relatively large fatty cholesterol chunks coated with protein are therefore called low-density lipoprotein, and they have a very nasty habit of not staying in the bloodstream. Instead, the LDLs dump off in any convenient arterial wall, enlarging the plaques we discussed earlier. On the other hand, the fat and cholesterol sometimes combine in tiny amounts, get coated with protein, and stay in the bloodstream very well indeed. These high-density lipoproteins even pick up some of the cholesterol that was dumped from the LDL and bring it back to the liver, where it can be eliminated. These HDL molecules seem to be the 'good guys' in the bloodstream. The fatty cholesterol plaques form inside the walls of the arteries when the cells of the walls get too filled up with LDL. The HDL actually blocks the cells' ability to ingest the LDL. You can see that it's to your advantage to have a high percentage of HDL and a low percentage of LDL. A man with a cholesterol reading of 250 milligrams percent but 80 percent LDL may be in more danger of arteriosclerosis than another man with 280 milligrams percent cholesterol but only 25 percent LDL.

Before menopause, women have a naturally high HDL, which helps to explain why they experience fewer heart attacks. Aerobic exercise also helps to elevate the HDL. Aerobic exercise has not definitely been shown to reduce total cholesterol levels, but it has been proved to increase the HDL percentage. It's not certain why this happens, but it looks as though the fat in the LDL is used to provide energy for the exercise, thus leaving a higher percentage of HDL.

If you eliminated all the cholesterol from your diet, would you then be able to get your blood cholesterol level to zero? Of course not! The amount of cholesterol you eat accounts for only part of the total cholesterol found in your body. Your liver produces a lot of cholesterol, an essential substance in the production of bile acids needed for the digestion of fat. In addition, cholesterol is the building block in the production of oestrogen and testosterone, the female and male sex hormones. Goodness knows what would happen if women and men didn't make oestrogen and testosterone – the whole world would go to pot! It's important for people to realize that cholesterol is a useful and necessary part of human life.

The raging argument, then, is whether you need to eat cholesterol at all. Most biochemists feel that your body would produce all the cholesterol it needs without getting any in the diet. As far as we know, the liver can make cholesterol out of any fat that you eat. But it will produce more cholesterol if you eat saturated fats and less cholesterol if you eat polyunsaturated fats. An interesting point is that the liver seems to produce more of the good HDL, and the dietary cholesterol contributes to more of the LDL. During a fast, however, the liver will produce more LDL. So, here again, is another reason to avoid radical or low-calorie dieting.

Please remember that fatty cholesterol deposits are influenced by the amount of cholesterol in the blood, but their formation is not solely dependent on it. Other factors, such as cigarette smoking and blood pressure, also play important roles. It's hard to prove that any one condition is responsible for arterial disease.

A patient who is put on a low-cholesterol diet by a doctor often feels overwhelmed by the lists of forbidden high-cholesterol foods. Eating from the bull's-eye of the Target is an easy way to maintain a low-cholesterol diet with no confusion. I would like you not only to limit the ingestion of fat and cholesterol, but to live a lifestyle that will make your body more competent to handle the amount of fat or cholesterol you do eat. Reduced sodium intake, more exercise, less stress, less overweight – these and other factors should all be combined in a total approach to health.

21

Try It – You'll Like It!

The Target Diet is not a diet! It's a way of looking at foods. It provides a technique for analysing what other people call diets. You can take any diet book, write down the foods it recommends for one day, and analyse it yourself. If you do this you will be shocked at how many diets violate the basic rules of good eating.

The Target approach doesn't forbid any food! If you must use butter, you can do it as long as your total number of fats for the day doesn't get out of hand. What constitutes getting out of hand? Well, it's different for different people. According to statistics, the average person gets 45 percent of his calories from fat, which is far too much. Very fit athletes can allow fat to contribute as much as 30 percent of their day's calories. If you are moderately fat and trying to reduce body fat stores, you shouldn't eat more than 20 percent fat calories. Obese people and those at high heart attack risk should keep dietary fat below 10 percent of total calories.

We all know that greasy, sugary foods are bad for us, but most of us don't do anything about it. The only way people change is when the decision comes from the inside – and no one can get inside you, except you. No doctor or dietitian or psychiatrist can change you – in spite of their exhortations to eat better, prescriptions of special diets, or the obvious wisdom of their advice. Entering your dietary habits into a computer with its impressive abilities won't change you either. The only thing that works is analysing your own diet. Forget the diet books and the big promises. You must do your own dietary analysis.

Keep in mind that the absolute accuracy of your dietary analysis is not the main point. The intent of this book, after all, is not to put professional dietitians out of business. It is to help you make healthy dietary adjustments, for which nothing is more effective than self-evaluation. Keep a record for a few days of everything you eat and drink. Then, using a Food Analysis sheet, analyse each day's intake by the Target method and decide for yourself if you are getting enough nutritious food without too much fat, sugar or alcohol. Believe me, when you analyse your diet yourself, it's a pretty powerful treatment, and you will make changes. Continue to analyse your diet periodically to keep tabs on your progress.

If I analyse your diet for you it won't work. An old proverb says, 'Feed a man a fish, and you feed him for a day. Teach a man how to fish, and you feed him for a lifetime'. The analysis sheets are not covered by copyright law. Please cut one out and Xerox as many copies as you wish. Share them with your friends. Walk through this book with your children and let them make their own changes. Instead of preaching to your kids, you will be teaching them how to fish – and it will feed them for a lifetime.

Good luck!

Appendix

The Target itself cannot possibly contain every known food. There simply isn't room to print them all on one piece of paper. The tables in this Appendix list far more foods than could be shown on the Target while giving the same information. The explanation for using these tables is on page 67.

Note that the amount of fat or sugar in a food may be slightly different in the tables from that shown on the Target. The reason for this is that quantities have to be rounded off a bit to fit the constraints of the Target. The numbers in the tables are slightly more accurate. A lot of judgment is required in estimating serving sizes, but rounding off figures will not make dietary analysis less valuable.

Extras

The foods listed in the Extras table are so lacking in vitamins, minerals, and protein that they don't deserve to be called foods. At best, we might call them empty-calorie foods. They shouldn't be printed on the Target because they are almost nutrition-free.

Fats: Each item under 'Fats', in the quantity shown, is one fat (5 5 grams of fat = 45 calories) in the Target system.
Sugars: Each item under 'Sugars', in the quantity shown, is one sugar in the Target system. This is approximately 11.5 grams of sugar and 45 calories. Note: A *teaspoon* of grease equals one fat or 45 calories. A *tablespoon* of sugar equals one sugar or 45 calories.
Alcohols: Each item under 'Alcohols', in the quantity shown, is called one alcohol in the Target system and contains approximately 105 calories.

Fats

1 teaspoon butter
1 teaspoon margarine
1 teaspoon vegetable oil
1 teaspoon bacon fat
1 teaspoon lard
1 teaspoon mayonnaise
½ tablespoon salad dressing
1 tablespoon top of the milk
1 tablespoon double cream
2 tablespoons single cream
2 tablespoons soured cream
¾-inch (2-cm) cube salt pork
1 tablespoon hollandaise sauce
1 teaspoon tartare sauce
1¼ tablespoons white sauce
2 tablespoons gravy

Sugars

1 tablespoon sugar
1 tablespoon icing sugar
1 tablespoon brown sugar
¾ tablespoon honey

1 tablespoon treacle or molasses
1 tablespoon syrup (golden, maple, chocolate)
1 tablespoon sauce (lemon, custard, caramel, butterscotch)
1¼ tablespoons jams, jellies, preserves
2 tablespoons cocoa mix, chocolate powder
⅓ oz (10 g) most sweets
4 fl oz (120 ml) soft drinks

Alcohols

1⅔ fl oz (50 ml) gin, rum, vodka, whisky
8 fl oz (250 ml) beer or ale
4 fl oz (120 ml) champagne or table wines
2 fl oz (60 ml) sherry or dessert wines

Meat Group

* = Add 100 calories
** = Subtract 40 calories
† = Not enough nutrients to justify one serving

	Target Units	
	Fat	Fibre
Beans, Peas and Lentils		
Black-eyed peas, 7 oz (200 g)*	¼	5
Garbanzo or Chick Peas, 7 oz (200 g)*	½	5
Kidney, 7 oz (200 g)*	¼	5
Lentils, 8 oz (225 g)*	0	5
Haricot, 8 oz (225 g)*	¼	5
Pinto, 7 oz (200 g)*	¼	5
Split peas, 8 oz (225 g)*	¼	5
White, 7 oz (200 g)*	¼	5
Beef		
Chuck, minced, 3½ oz (100 g)	5	
Chuck, lean only, 3½ oz (100 g)	2	
Corned, 3½ oz (100 g)	6	
Heart, 3½ oz (100 g)	1	
Liver, 3½ oz (100 g)	1	
Minced, lean, 10% fat, 3½ oz (100 g)	2	
Minced, 21% fat, 3½ oz (100 g)	3½	
Roast, rib, lean and fat, 3½ oz (100 g)	7½	
Roast, rib, lean only, 3½ oz (100 g)	2½	
Roast, silverside, lean and fat, 3½ oz (100 g)	5	
Roast, silverside, lean only, 3½ oz (100 g)	2	
Roast, top side, 3½ oz (100 g)	2	
Steak, flank, 3½ oz (100 g)	1½	
Steak, porterhouse, 3½ oz (100 g)	1½	
Steak, sirloin, 3½ oz (100 g)	1½	
Steak, T-bone, 3½ oz (100 g)	2	
Steak, fillet, 3½ oz (100 g)	2	
Steak, rump 3½ oz (100 g)	1	
Tongue, 3½ oz (100 g)	2	
Tripe, 3½ oz (100 g)	½	

	Target Units	
	Fat	Fibre
Fish and Seafood		
Cod, 4½ oz (130 g)**	⅕	
Crab, 4½ oz (130 g)	⅓	
Haddock, 4½ oz (130 g)**	⅕	
Halibut, 4½ oz (130 g)	⅓	
Herring, 4½ oz (130 g)	⅓	
Lobster, 4½ oz (130 g)	⅓	
Mackerel, 3½ oz (100 g)	2	
Oysters, 4½ oz (130 g)	⅓	
Perch, 4½ oz (130 g)	⅓	
Plaice, 4½ oz (130 g)**	⅕	
Prawns, 4½ oz (130 g)	¼	
Rock salmon 4½ oz (130 g)	⅔	
Salmon, red, 3½ oz (100 g)	2½	
Salmon, pink, 4½ oz (130 g)	1	
Sardines, in oil, 8 medium	5	
Scallops, 4½ oz (130 g)	¼	
Sole, 4½ oz (130 g)**	⅕	
Trout, river, 4½ oz (130 g)	½	
Trout, rainbow, 3½ oz (100 g)	2	
Tuna, in oil, 3 oz (75 g)	1½	
Tuna, in water, 3 oz (75 g)	⅓	
Game and Speciality Meats		
Duck, domestic, 3½ oz (100 g)	4½	
Duck, wild, 3½ oz (100 g)	1	
Frogs' legs, 3½ oz (100 g)**	0	
Goose, 3½ oz (100 g)	2	
Pheasant, 3½ oz (100 g)	1	
Quail, 3½ oz (100 g)	1½	
Rabbit, 3½ oz (100 g)	1	
Venison, 3½ oz (100 g)	½	
Lamb		
Cutlets, lean and fat, 3½ oz (100 g)	4	
Cutlets, lean only, 3½ oz (100 g)	1½	
Leg, lean and fat, 3½ oz (100 g)	3	
Leg, lean only, 3½ oz (100 g)	1	
Loin chop, lean and fat, 3½ oz (100 g)	3	
Loin chop, lean only 3½ oz (100 g)	1	

134

Nuts and Seeds

	Fat	Fibre
Almonds, 4 oz (115 g)(½ meat) †	11	1½
Cashews, 3 oz (75 g)	5½	1½
Chestnuts, 6 oz (175 g)	½	1½
Coconut, 2 oz (50 g)(½ meat) †	4½	1
Macadamia nuts, 3 oz (75 g)(½ meat) †	9½	1½
Peanut butter, 2 tablespoons (½ meat) †	3	½
Peanuts, 4 oz (115 g)	5½	1½
Pecans, 3 oz (75 g) (½ meat) †	9	1½
Pine nuts, 3 oz (75 g)	8	1½
Pistachios, 3 oz (75 g)	7	1½
Pumpkin seeds, 3 oz (75 g)	5½	1½
Sunflower seeds 3 oz (75 g)	5½	1½
Walnuts, 3 oz (75 g) (½ meat) †	9	1½

Pork

	Fat	Fibre
Bacon, 6 rashers**	3½	
Back bacon, 3½ oz (100 g)	3	
Chop, lean only, 3½ oz (100 g)	2½	
Ham, lean and fat, 3½ oz (100 g)	5½	
Ham, lean only, 3½ oz (100 g)	2	
Ham, picnic, lean only, 3½ oz (100 g)	2	
Sausages, 3	5	
Sausage meat 3½ oz (100 g)	6	
Spareribs, 3–4 small	4	

Poultry

	Fat	Fibre
Chicken and turkey, dark meat, no skin, 3½ oz (100 g)	1½	
Chicken and turkey, white meat, no skin, 3½ oz (100 g)	½	
Chicken and turkey, white or dark meat with skin, 3½ oz (100 g)	3	

Veal

	Fat	Fibre
Best end neck, 3½ oz (100 g)	1	
Escalope, 3½ oz (100 g)	3	
Fillet, 3½ oz (100 g)	1½	
Loin, 3½ oz (100 g)	1	
Shoulder, 3½ oz (100 g)	1	
Stew, lean and fat, 3½ oz (100 g)	5	

	Target Units	
	Fat	**Fibre**
Miscellaneous and Luncheon Meats		
Bologna, 4 slices	6½	
Eggs, 2**	2	
Hot dogs, 2**	4	
Knockwurst, 3½ oz (100 g)**	4½	
Liverwurst, 3½ oz (100 g)	6½	
Pepperoni, 3½ oz (100 g)	9	
Salami, 3 slices	3	
Sausage, Polish, 3 slices**	4	
Sausage, salami, 3½ oz (100 g)	6½	
Spam, 3½ oz (100 g)	5	
Tofu, 3½ oz (100 g) (½ meat) †	1	

Milk Group

** = Subtract 40 calories

	Target Units	
	Fat	Sugar
Milk		
Buttermilk, from skimmed, 8 fl oz (250 ml)	0	
Buttermilk, from whole, 8 fl oz (250 ml)	½	
Chocolate (1% fat), 8 fl oz (250 ml)	½	1⅓
Chocolate (2% fat), 8 fl oz (250 ml)	1	1⅓
Coconut, 8 fl oz (250 ml)	12	
Evaporated, 4 fl oz (120 ml)	1½	
Low-fat (1%), 8 fl oz (250 ml)	½	
Low-fat (2%), 8 fl oz (250 ml)	1	
Skimmed, 8 fl oz (250 ml)	0	
Whole (3.5% fat), 8 fl oz (250 ml)	1⅔	
Cheese		
Blue, 1⅓ oz (35 g)**	2⅓	
Brie, 1⅓ oz (35 g)**	2	
Camembert, 1⅓ oz (35 g)**	1⅔	
Cheddar, 1⅓ oz (35 g)**	2½	
Cottage, full-fat, 4 oz (115 g)	1	
Cottage, low-fat, 4 oz (115 g)	¼	
Cream, 2½ tablespoons (does not count as a milk serving; nutrients are too low)	2½	
Feta, 1⅓ oz (35 g)**	1½	
Gouda, 1⅓ oz (35 g)**	2	
Gruyère, 1⅓ oz (35 g)**	2⅓	
Mozzarella, 1⅓ oz (35 g)**	1½	
Neufchâtel, 1⅓ oz (35 g) (does not count as a milk serving; nutrients are too low)	1½	
Provolone, 1⅓ oz (35 g)**	2	
Ricotta, 4 oz (115 g)	3	
Roquefort, 1⅓ oz (35 g)**	2⅓	
Swiss, 1⅓ oz (35 g)**	2	
Cheese spreads, 1⅓ oz (35 g)**	1½	
Dessert		
Ice cream, 6 oz (175 g)	4⅓	2½

Yoghurt
Low-fat, fruit-flavoured, ¼ pint (150 ml)   ½   1½
Low-fat, plain, ¼ pint (150 ml)   ½

Fruit and Vegetable Group

| | Target Units | | |
	Fat	Fibre	Sugar
Fruits			
Apple, 1 small, whole		1	
Apricot, 2 medium, raw		1	
Apricots, dried, 3 oz (75 g)		2	2
Avocado, ½ medium	3½	3	
Banana, ½ small		1	
Blackberries, 3 oz (75 g)		5	
Blueberries, 2 oz (50 g)		2	
Cantaloupe, ¼ melon		1	
Cherries, red, 2 oz (50 g)		1	
Cranberries, 4 oz (100 g)		2	
Dates, 10 medium		4	6
Figs, 2 small		1	
Figs, dried, 4 medium		7	5
Grapefruit, ½ medium		1	
Grapes, seedless, 2 oz (50 g)		1	
Honeydew, ¼ small		1	
Mango, ½ medium		1½	
Nectarine, 1 medium		1	
Olives, green, 6 medium	2	1	
Orange, 1 small		2	
Papaya, ⅓ medium		1½	
Peach, 1 medium		1	
Peaches, dried, 3 oz (75 g)		4	5
Pear, ½ medium		2	
Pineapple, 3 oz (75 g)		1	
Plums, 2 small		1	
Prunes, 8 large		4	8
Raisins, 3 oz (75 g)		1½	6
Raspberries, 3 oz (75 g)		3	
Rhubarb, 4 oz (100 g)		1	

| | Target Units | | |
	Fat	Fibre	Sugar
Strawberries, 10 large		2	
Strawberries, frozen sliced, sweet, 3 oz (75 g)		2	2
Tangerine, 1 large		1	
Watermelon, 4 oz (100 g)		1	

Vegetables

Artichoke, 1 medium		4	
Asparagus, 5–6 spears		1	
Aubergine, 4 oz (115 g)		1	
Beans, green, 6 oz (175 g)		2	
Beetroot, 4 oz (115 g)		1	
Broccoli, 6 oz (175 g)		3	
Brussels sprouts, 9 medium		3	
Cabbage, 8 oz (225 g)		2	
Cabbage, red, 4 oz (115 g)		2	
Carrot, 1 large		2	
Cauliflower, 4 oz (115 g)		2	
Celery, 4 oz (115 g)		2	
Cucumber, 1 medium		1	
Lettuce, iceberg		2	
Mushrooms, 4 oz (115 g)		2	
Okra, 8–9 pods		2	
Onions, 4 oz (115 g)		2	
Peas, 3 oz (75 g)		2	
Potato, ½ medium		1	
Spinach, 3 oz (75 g)		2	
Sweet potato, 1 small		1	2
Tomato, 1 large		2	

Juices and Juice Drinks

Apple juice, 4 fl oz (120 ml)		½	½

Target Units

	Fat	Fibre	Sugar
Apricot juice, 4 fl oz (120 ml)		½	½
Carrot juice, 4 fl oz (120 ml)		½	½
Grapefruit juice, 4 fl oz (120 ml)		½	½
Grape juice, 4 fl oz (120 ml)			1
Grape juice drink, 4 fl oz (120 ml)			½
Guava juice, 4 fl oz (120 ml)		½	1
Lemonade, 4 fl oz (120 ml)			½
Orange juice, 4 fl oz (120 ml)		½	½
Papaya juice, 4 fl oz (120 ml)		½	1
Pineapple juice, 4 fl oz (120 ml)		½	½
Prune juice, 4 fl oz (120 ml)		½	1
Tomato juice, 4 fl oz (120 ml)		½	
Tomato juice cocktail, 4 fl oz (120 ml)		½	

Bread and Cereal Group

| | Target Units | | |
	Fat	Fibre	Sugar
Breads			
Bagel, ½	⅓	½	
Corn bread, 1 piece	1	1	
French, 1 slice		½	
Italian, 1 slice		½	
Pumpernickel, 1 slice		2	
Rye, 1 slice		2	
Scone, 1	1⅓	½	
White, 1 slice		½	
Wholemeal, 1 slice		2	
Bread sticks, 3 average		½	
Buns			
Hamburger, ½		½	
Hot dog, ½		½	
Cakes			
Angel, 1 piece, ¹/₁₂ cake			1
Brownie, 1 piece	2		1
Carrot, 1 piece, ¹/₁₂ cake	2		1
Cheesecake, 1 piece, ¹/₁₂ cake	3		1
Chocolate, 1 piece, ¹/₁₂ cake	2		1
Cupcake, 1	1		1
Fruitcake, 1 piece, ¹/₁₂ cake	1		1
Gingerbread, 1 piece, ¹/₁₂ cake	1		1
Madeira, 1 piece, ¹/₁₂ cake	1½		
Spice, 1 piece, ¹/₁₂ cake	1		1
Sponge, Genoese, 1 piece, ¹/₁₂ cake	½		
Sponge, sandwich cake, 1 piece, ¹/₁₂ cake	1½		1
Cereals			
Bran Cereals			
Kellogg's All-Bran, 1 oz (25 g)		9	½
Kellogg's Bran Buds, 1 oz (25 g)		8	⅔
Kellogg's 40% Bran Flakes, 1 oz (25 g)		4	½
Raisin Bran 1 oz (25 g)		4	1

	Target Units		
	Fat	Fibre	Sugar
Cold Cereals			
Grape-nuts, 1 oz (25 g)		2	1/3
Puffed Rice, 2 oz (50 g)		1	0
Puffed Wheat, 2 oz (50 g)		2	0
Shredded Wheat, 1 biscuit		4	0
Muesli, 1 oz (25 g)		2	1/3
Hot Cereals			
Quaker Oats, 1 oz (25 g)		1	0
Sugared Cereals, 1 oz (25 g)		1/2	2
Wheat Germ, 1 oz (25 g)	1/2	0	0
Crisps			
Corn chips, 1 oz (25 g)	2	1/2	
Potato, 1 oz (25 g)	1 1/2	1/2	
Tortilla chips, 1 oz (25 g)	1 1/2	1/2	
Crackers etc			
Cheese savoury biscuits, bite-size			
20 pieces	1/2	1/2	
Digestive, 3	1/3	1/2	
Ritz, 6 pieces	1	1/2	
Crispbread, 4 pieces	0	1/2	
Cream crackers, 6 pieces	1/2	1/2	
Biscuits			
Butter, 4	1/2		
Chocolate chip, 4	2 1/2		1
Coconut macaroons, 2	1		1
Oatmeal, 2	1 1/2	1/2	1
Peanut butter, 2	1		1/2
Vanilla wafers, 6	1/2		1/2
Doughnuts			
Cream-filled, 1	1		1/2
Chocolate-covered, 1	3		2
Plain, 1	1		1/2

	Target Units		
	Fat	**Fibre**	**Sugar**
Muffins			
Bran, 1	$2/3$	1	
English, $1/2$	$1/3$	$1/2$	
English, wholemeal, $1/2$	$1/3$	1	
Wholemeal, 1	$1/3$	$1/2$	
Pasta			
Macaroni, cooked, 2 oz (50 g)		$1/2$	
Macaroni, wholemeal, cooked, 2 oz (50 g)		1	
Noodles, egg, cooked, 2 oz (50 g)	$1/3$	$1/2$	
Spaghetti, cooked, 2 oz (50 g)		$1/2$	
Spaghetti, wholemeal, cooked, 2 oz (50 g)		1	
Pies			
Cream, 1 serving or $1/7$	3		4
Fruit, 1 serving or $1/7$	3		2
Rice			
Brown, $2\frac{1}{2}$ oz (65 g) cooked		1	
White, $2\frac{1}{2}$ oz (65 g) cooked		$1/2$	
Wild, $2\frac{1}{2}$ oz (65 g) cooked		2	
Miscellaneous			
Pancake, 1	$1/2$	$1/2$	
Pretzels, 2 average	$1/3$	$1/2$	
Stuffing, 4 oz (115 g)	3	1	
Tortilla, corn, 1		2	
Tortilla, flour, 1	$1/2$	$1/2$	
Tortilla, whole-wheat flour, 1		2	
Waffle, $1/2$ section	$1/2$	$1/2$	

Combination Foods, Fast Foods, and Soups

* = add 100 calories to Meat Group
** = subtract 40 calories from Milk Group

	Servings				Target Units		
	Meat	Milk	F&V	B&C	Fibre	Fat	Sugar
Combination Foods							
Beans and frankfurters, canned, 6 oz (175 g)	1				2	3	
Beef stew, canned, 8 oz (225 g)	½		1		1	1	
Cabbage rolls, stuffed, 2 average	½		1		1	2	
Cheese macaroni, frozen, 8 oz (225 g)**		1		2	1	2	
Chicken à la king, frozen, 1 package	1		½		1	3	
Chili, vegetarian, 8 oz (225 g)	1				5	¼	
Chili con carne, canned, 8 oz (225 g)*	1				5	4	
Chow mein, chicken, frozen, 1 package	1		½		1	1	
Fish cakes, fried, frozen, 2	1					3½	
Lasagna, frozen, 1 package**	½	1	¼	1	½	3	
Macaroni and beef, frozen, 1 package	½			1	½	2	
Pizza, cheese, 1 piece**		1		1	½	1	
Pizza with pepperoni, 1 piece**	¼	1		1	½	2	
Pizza with sausage, 1 piece**	¼	1		1	½	2	
Ravioli, canned, 4 fl oz (120 ml)	½			1	½	2	
Spaghetti sauce, 4 fl oz (120 ml)			½			1½	
Spaghetti sauce with meat, 4 fl oz (120 ml)	¼		½			1½	
Taco, 1 average	½	¼	¼	1	½	1½	
Tostada, 1	½	¼	¼		1	1½	
Fast Foods							
Cheeseburger, small	¾	½(-20)		2	1	2½	
Cheeseburger, large**	1	1		2	1	3½	
Chips or french fries, about 6 oz (175 g)			1		½	4	
Cole slaw, 4 oz (115 g)				1	2	1½	

145

	Servings				Target Units		
	Meat	Milk	F&V	B&C	Fibre	Fat	Sugar
Fish, fried, 1 piece	1					4	
Fish sandwich	1			2	1	4	
Hamburger	¾			2	1	2½	
Hamburger, large	1			2	1	3½	
Popcorn, 2 oz (50 g) (no food group; add 50 calories)					1		
Shake, vanilla or chocolate		1				3	2½

Soups (canned)

	Meat	Milk	F&V	B&C	Fibre	Fat	Sugar
Asparagus, cream of, 8 fl oz (250 ml)		1	¼		½	2	
Bean, 8 fl oz (250 ml)*					5	1	
Beef or chicken broth, bouillon, or consommé (no food group; add 40 calories for 8 fl oz (250 ml))							
Beef noodle, 8 fl oz (250 ml)	½			1	½	½	
Celery, cream of, with milk, 8 fl oz (250 ml)		1	¼		½	½	
Cheddar cheese, 8 fl oz (250 ml)**		1				2	
Chicken, cream of, with milk, 8 fl oz (250 ml)		1				2	
Chicken noodle, 8 fl oz (250 ml)				1	½	½	
Fish chowder, 8 fl oz (250 ml)	¼	½	½			1	
Minestrone, 8 fl oz (250 ml)			1		4	½	
Mushroom, cream of, with milk, 8 fl oz (250 ml)		1	¼			2	
Onion, 8 fl oz (250 ml)			½		½	½	
Oyster stew, 8 fl oz (250 ml)	¼		½		½	2	
Pea green, 8 fl oz (250 ml)			1		2	½	
Pea split, 8 fl oz (250 ml)	1				5	½	
Potato, 8 fl oz (250 ml)		1	1		1	1½	
Tomato, 8 fl oz (250 ml)			1		1	½	
Vegetable, 8 fl oz (250 ml)			1		1	½	

The Target Diet Food Analysis Sheet (Please feel free to make copies of this page)

Instructions on page 61

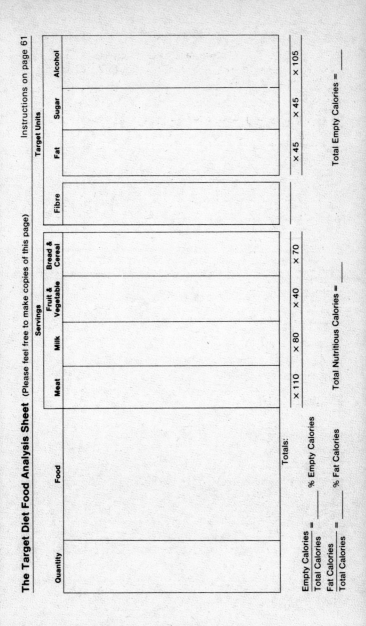

Quantity	Food	Servings				Target Units			
		Meat	Milk	Fruit & Vegetable	Bread & Cereal	Fibre	Fat	Sugar	Alcohol

Totals:

× 110   × 80   × 40   × 70   × 45   × 45   × 105

Total Nutritious Calories = _____   Total Empty Calories = _____

Empty Calories = _____ % Empty Calories
Total Calories

Fat Calories = _____ % Fat Calories
Total Calories

The Target Diet Food Analysis Sheet (Please feel free to make copies of this page)

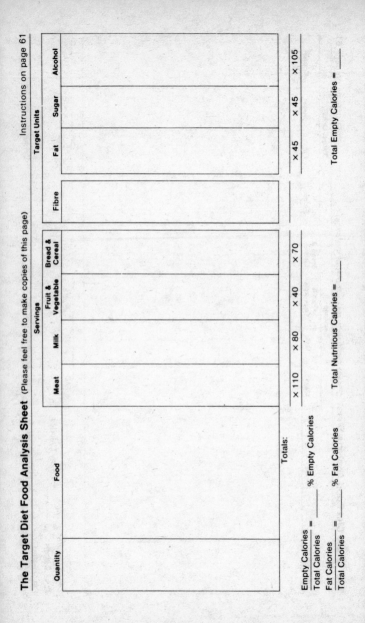

Instructions on page 61

Quantity	Food	Servings					Target Units			
		Meat	Milk	Fruit & Vegetable	Bread & Cereal	Fibre	Fat	Sugar	Alcohol
Totals:		× 110	× 80	× 40	× 70		× 45	× 45	× 105
		Total Nutritious Calories = _____					Total Empty Calories = _____		

Empty Calories = _____ % Empty Calories
Total Calories

Fat Calories = _____ % Fat Calories
Total Calories

The Target Diet Food Analysis Sheet (Please feel free to make copies of this page)

Instructions on page 61

Quantity	Food	Servings				Target Units			
		Meat	Milk	Fruit & Vegetable	Bread & Cereal	Fibre	Fat	Sugar	Alcohol

	× 110	× 80	× 40	× 70		× 45	× 45	× 105
Totals:								

Total Nutritious Calories = _____   Total Empty Calories = _____

$$\frac{\text{Empty Calories}}{\text{Total Calories}} = _____ \text{ \% Empty Calories}$$

$$\frac{\text{Fat Calories}}{\text{Total Calories}} = _____ \text{ \% Fat Calories}$$

The Target Diet Food Analysis Sheet (Please feel free to make copies of this page)

Instructions on page 61

Quantity	Food	Meat	Milk	Fruit & Vegetable	Bread & Cereal	Fibre	Fat	Sugar	Alcohol
	Totals:								
		× 110	× 80	× 40	× 70		× 45	× 45	× 105
		Total Nutritious Calories = _____					Total Empty Calories = _____		

Servings

Target Units

Empty Calories / Total Calories = _____ % Empty Calories

Fat Calories / Total Calories = _____ % Fat Calories

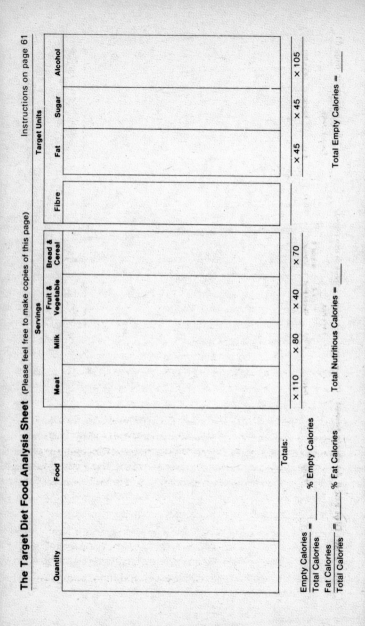

The Target Diet Food Analysis Sheet (Please feel free to make copies of this page)

Instructions on page 61

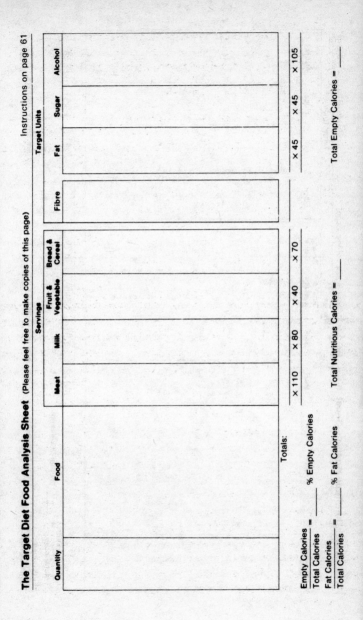

Quantity	Food	Meat	Milk	Fruit & Vegetable	Bread & Cereal	Fibre	Fat	Sugar	Alcohol

Totals:

× 110 × 80 × 40 × 70 × 45 × 45 × 105

Total Nutritious Calories = _____

Total Empty Calories = _____

Empty Calories = _____ % Empty Calories

Total Calories

Fat Calories = _____ % Fat Calories

Total Calories

The Target Diet Food Analysis Sheet (Please feel free to make copies of this page)

Instructions on page 61

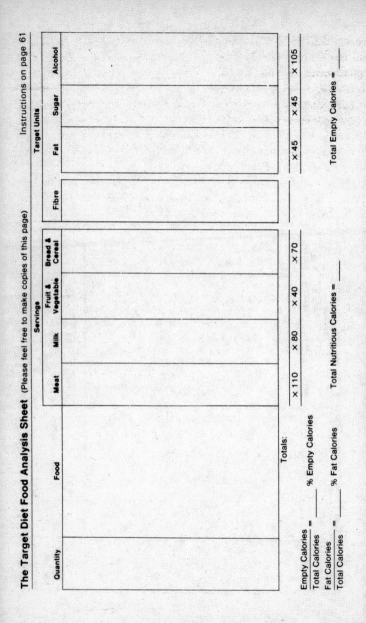

Quantity	Food	Servings				Fibre	Target Units		
		Meat	Milk	Fruit & Vegetable	Bread & Cereal		Fat	Sugar	Alcohol
	Totals:								
		× 110	× 80	× 40	× 70		× 45	× 45	× 105
		Total Nutritious Calories = ____					Total Empty Calories =		

$$\frac{\text{Empty Calories}}{\text{Total Calories}} = \underline{\quad\quad} \text{\% Empty Calories}$$

$$\frac{\text{Fat Calories}}{\text{Total Calories}} = \underline{\quad\quad} \text{\% Fat Calories}$$